CIRCUMCISION AND MEDICINE
IN MODERN TURKEY

CIRCUMCISION AND MEDICINE IN MODERN TURKEY

OYMAN BAŞARAN

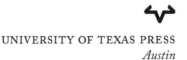

UNIVERSITY OF TEXAS PRESS
Austin

Requests for permission to reproduce material from this work should be sent to:
Permissions
University of Texas Press
P.O. Box 7819
Austin, TX 78713-7819
utpress.utexas.edu/rp-form

♾ The paper used in this book meets the minimum requirements of
ANSI/NISO Z39.48-1992 (R1997) (Permanence of Paper).

LIBRARY OF CONGRESS CATALOGING-IN-PUBLICATION DATA

Names: Başaran, Oyman, author.
Title: Circumcision and medicine in modern Turkey / Oyman Başaran.
Description: First edition. | Austin : University of Texas Press, 2023. | Includes
bibliographical references and index.
Identifiers: LCCN 2022017160 (print) | LCCN 2022017161 (ebook)
  ISBN 978-1-4773-2702-9 (hardcover)
  ISBN 978-1-4773-2703-6 (pdf)
  ISBN 978-1-4773-2704-3 (epub)
Subjects: LCSH: Circumcision—Turkey—History—20th century. |
Circumcision—Turkey—History—21st century. | Circumcision—Social
aspects—Turkey. | Medical personnel—Turkey—Social conditions. |
Circumcision—Political aspects—Turkey.
Classification: LCC GN484 .B36 2023 (print) | LCC GN484 (ebook) |
DDC 392.109561/0904—dc23/eng/20220525
LC record available at https://lccn.loc.gov/2022017160
LC ebook record available at https://lccn.loc.gov/2022017161

doi:10.7560/327029

CONTENTS

ACKNOWLEDGMENTS

This book would not have emerged without the support of many colleagues, friends, and family. I embarked on this project during my years as a doctoral student at the University of Massachusetts, Amherst. I owe thanks to my advisor, Janice Irvine, for her continued guidance and to my dissertation committee members, Fareen Parvez and Christopher T. Dole, for their helpful comments on earlier versions of the book.

I am indebted to all my colleagues in sociology at Bowdoin College: Nancy E. Riley, Shruti Devgan, Marcos Lopez, Ingrid A. Nelson, Theodore Greene, and Lori Brackett. My special thanks go to Nancy and Ingrid for their excellent mentorship and support. I thank Nancy for her insightful feedback on my book as well.

My writing group with Shenila (Khoja-Moolji), Shruti (Devgan), and Jay (Sosa) has been extremely generative. They have read different iterations of each chapter and provided very valuable feedback on them. Their patience and sustained support and friendship helped me tremendously as I made my way through the maze of the writing process.

I would like to thank my editor, Jim Burr, for his support of the project. My gratitude goes to Can Açıksöz, Roi Livne, and Kelly Joyce, as well as the University of Texas Press anonymous reviewer, for their constructive criticism and insightful suggestions.

I want to thank several people who shaped my thinking long before I began this project: Meltem Ahıska, Nükhet Sirman, Nazan Üstündağ, Suna Ertuğrul, Gürol Irzık, and Ferda Keskin. I am also very grateful to my friends for their support and kindness: Bengi (Akbulut), Aslı, Aycan, Emir, Bengi (Baran), Meryem, Willi, Değer, Can, Simon, Swati, Adanna, Sebastian, and Salar.

I couldn't have written this book without my family's support. Thank you to my parents, my sister, my in-laws, and Liam. My sister, Pelin, has always been my confidant and my source of strength. Taking long walks daily with our loving little furry friend, Flóki, and watching him chase butterflies have kept my sanity during the writing process. My deepest gratitude goes to Alyssa for her unflagging love, endless support, and being a close intellectual interlocutor.

I dedicate this book to my mother, whose insatiable curiosity exceeded what life was ready to offer her.

I was circumcised at the age of eight. It was a summer day, the typical season for male circumcisions in Turkey. Our apartment in Istanbul was crowded with neighbors and relatives, and since my father had told me that I would not be circumcised until the next day, I did not quite understand why we had people over then. A few days before the gathering, my mother had asked me to put on a circumcision outfit that made me look like a little "sultan" and had taken me to visit neighbors, relatives, and a shrine, the first phase of a circumcision ritual that usually spreads over several days. At the shrine, I saw dozens of other boys around my age who were wearing similar circumcision outfits and praying with their parents. Like all rituals, the circumcision ritual in Turkey has a strong communal dimension that highlights the role of an audience in witnessing and affirming what is supposed to be a milestone in a boy's life, hence the importance of our visits. Taken together, the visits, the carefully selected clothing, and the prayers rendered that summer different from an ordinary summer. These ritual elements initiated, as I was told, my first step in the passage from boyhood to manhood.

Circumcision was for me a nebulous event surrounded by uncertainties, as I didn't know what to expect. That day, as friends and family gathered in our apartment, my father noticed my confusion and frustration. He told me a sünnetçi (circumciser) would come over in the afternoon—just for a checkup, he assured me—and would not circumcise me until the next day. Meanwhile, our female neighbors and relatives were in the kitchen, cooking and preparing food, and the men were sitting and talking in the living room. The sünnetçi, who was also a health officer, finally arrived alone. He had me sit on the couch in the living room. I was wearing my circumcision outfit. The sünnetçi asked me to pull down my shorts and underwear. He injected my groin with what I now know was an anesthetic, commonly used by health officers. He then told me that he just wanted to check my penis. Within a few minutes, my penis felt numbed and the men in the room had me lie down on the dining table, which had been covered with a sheet. I was surrounded by my father, my two uncles, and my grandfather—all were holding down my arms. The women, including my mother, stayed in the kitchen, and I could hear some of them praying. The sünnetçi came to the table and took his instruments out of his black bag. The next thing I remember is the circumciser's smiling face as he showed me my foreskin, now hanging from a pair of scissors. I was surprised. The women joined us in the living room, everyone clapping and congratulating me on my bravery.

My younger cousin was also circumcised on the same day. Families often have brothers or male cousins close to each other in age circumcised at the same time to reduce the costs of both the operation (circumcisers charge less for the second boy) and the requisite celebration. Afterward, the celebration moved to a wedding hall.[1] There, my cousin and I, again in our circumcision outfits, were placed on a decorated bed in the center of the hall to recuperate. We covered our newly circumcised and sutured penises with our fez-like blue hats, a common practice to protect the penis from being bumped or jostled during recovery. Relatives and neighbors took pictures of us and posed for photos with us. "Girls should be scared," they told us, "since we were now men." Some adult men asked mischievously to peek at our circumcised penises or asked us to show them, another circumcision-related practice common in Turkey. A (newly) circumcised penis is considered acceptable for semipublic display, and boys are expected to want to show it off. Food and drinks were served. In the evening, an imam came to our apartment to recite religious poems with the relatives and neighbors present.

The operation itself was not painful, but I remember being worried about it before and after the event. In the days leading up to the ceremony, my peers and some young adult men made jokes about circumcision (for example, that the circumciser was going to cut off my penis with an ax), which put me on edge, to say the least, even though I knew at some level that it wasn't true. Later, compared to my cousin's recovery, my recovery was long and painful due to inflammation. With the help of my mother, I applied antibiotic ointment to the inflamed incision and dressed it a couple of times daily until, finally, it healed as a scab.

Pain and fear of pain were central to my experience of male circumcision: my parents kept the actual date of the operation secret in the hopes that I would not panic, the sünnetçi applied local anesthetic so that I would not feel pain, the adult men held me tight during the operation in case I felt pain or became frightened and flailed too much (which could jeopardize the safety of the procedure for both the circumciser and me), and I was praised and given gifts for braving the operation without crying. Whether or not we said so openly, we all considered male circumcision as a potentially painful operation that caused concern and required appropriate mitigation.

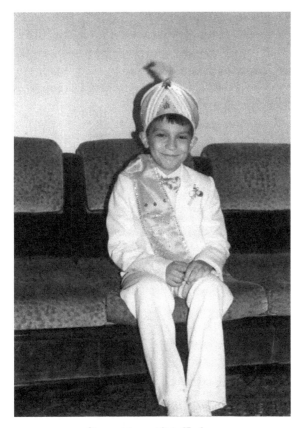

Circumcision outfit in Turkey

My 1980s circumcision was not exception when it comes to mitigating circumcision pain in Turkey. Every year, thousands of boys in Turkey undergo circumcision operations where families and circumcisers alike take great care carrying out the procedure without causing pain for boys. Circumcisers, boys, and families generally see circumcision pain in multiple forms: dread of the procedure, the immediate pain caused by cutting off the foreskin (in the absence of anesthesia), risk of excessive and potentially fatal blood loss, long recovery, and trauma.

Sünnetçi is a term charged with conflicting sentiments and meanings in Turkey: a cause of fear for young boys, a specter of punishment that families may invoke to discipline their sons, and an identity that medical professionals assume—or reject—often with a gnawing sense of unease. He represents as much an embarrassing relic of the past and an obstacle to progress as a promise of a healthy society and consumer comfort. Medical actors—for instance, the health officer who circumcised me—have, over the long twentieth century and up to the present day, increasingly become involved with male circumcision in Turkey, and their involvement, situated in changing health care infrastructures, has reshaped how circumcision pain is managed and the role of the sünnetçi is understood. This transformation is the subject of this book.

SÜNNETÇİ, PAIN, AND MEDICINE

Recognition is the misrecognition you can bear, a transaction that affirms you without . . . necessarily feeling good or being accurate.

LAURENT BERLANT, *CRUEL OPTIMISM* (BERLANT 2011, P. 26)

"At first, I did not want to start performing circumcision," Necmi said.[1] A sixty-five-year-old health officer, Necmi was part of a health care network that, from the 1960s onwards, spread across the country. After middle school, he was trained in medicine and public health at a state-funded vocational medical school (sağlık koleji). After graduating at the top of the class, he completed a year and a half of mandatory military service, where he assisted a doctor with circumcision operations. The Ministry of Health then assigned him to a town in the Central Anatolia Region of Turkey.[2] Necmi, along with other health officers, introduced local anesthesia and suture to prevent pain during and after the operation and usually circumcised boys at their homes. Like his colleagues, he wanted to drive his competitors, the itinerant circumcisers who had been serving locals for generations even though a law passed in 1928 banned them from the practice, out of business. For Necmi, the ban was justified because itinerant circumcisers' techniques, he believed, could harm boys.

Necmi was born in a village in western Turkey and his father had been a shepherd. "We were five siblings and were very poor," he said. An itinerant circumciser circumcised Necmi at a young age at his village: "some kids tried to run away when the circumciser came to our village," he said, smiling. "But I wanted to be circumcised," he added. Becoming a public employee was, unsurprisingly, a crucial opportunity for him (and other health officers) to extract himself from poverty and support his parents. I interviewed him at the home he had purchased with the additional income coming from performing circumcision for over twenty-five years. Granted, not all health officers I interviewed had fared as well as Necmi (though some did even better than him); they all nonetheless welcomed the supplementary income.

Thus, given his positive memories of his own circumcision and the financial opportunities circumcision provided, I was surprised to hear that Necmi had waited for several years before starting his practice. When I asked him about his reluctance, Necmi replied, "Itinerant circumcisers were doing it. I did not want to be mistaken for them. Also, you are working on a boy's most important organ. You can ruin their life." These were the reasons, he highlighted,

1

why his friend from the same medical school never performed circumcision. In the meantime, some of the senior itinerant circumcisers against whom he competed had learned to use surgical techniques as well. He explained that a doctor taught them so that they could better manage pain and postsurgical complications.

Necmi was living in the city center, and since the city was small, I was curious to know whether he went to villages for circumcision as well and, if he did, how he traveled around. My question upset him, as he thought that I was comparing him to itinerant circumcisers: "No, I am not like them [itinerant circumcisers]! I don't travel around." Still, like itinerant circumcisers, Necmi indeed went to villages for circumcision, but only by appointment and without staying overnight. Over time, itinerant circumcisers at the city had retired and Necmi became the only sünnetçi in the area with medical expertise.

Circumcision and Medicine in Modern Turkey examines the ways circumcisers, like the health officer Necmi, have, over the twentieth century and up to the present day, attached themselves to the medicalization process, thereby reshaping the techniques, goals, and discourses concerning male circumcision in Turkey. It makes two interrelated interventions. First, it enriches our sociological understanding of the medicalization process. The dominant view of medicalization in the public imagination and scholarly writings presumes a straightforward link between the actors of medicalization, whether they be medical professionals or Big Pharma, and the targets of medicalization. According to this view, medicalization is merely a tool and opportunity for actors to expand their power into new territory and further pursue their professional and economic interests. This view accepts medical actors' desires for medicalization as given.

However, based on this top-down view of medicalization, we would have a hard time making sense of Necmi's initial hesitancy or his friend's lack of interest in male circumcision despite its potential financial rewards. Necmi's affective investment in the medicalization of male circumcision was anything but a spontaneous and inevitable occurrence. Nor was it a logical outcome of his presumed preexisting economic and professional ambitions. His case thus suggests that, for a complete picture of the medicalization process, we need a better understanding of medical actors' subjectivity, of *how* and *why* they bind themselves to medicine. Accordingly, throughout *Circumcision and Medicine in Modern Turkey*, I will problematize circumcisers' desires to (continue to) invest in the medicalization of male circumcision in Turkey. I will show that along with the medicalization of male circumcision came changes in the subjectivity of circumcisers.

Second, the book's broader conceptual gesture emerges from a dissatisfaction with the dominant theories of subjectivity in sociology, ranging from labeling theory to social interactionism and phenomenological approaches. Sociology tends to formulate subjectivity as an effect of social facts (scripts, discourses, ideals, and norms), an effect produced via various operations such as internalization, inculcation, socialization, resistance, opposition, or reinscription, all of which can work on conscious and nonconscious levels. Yet, none of these heuristic tools, at least as they are usually formulated, can explain the affective grip of the social world on us and why we respond to social facts in the first place. The standard sociological answer to this question fails to rise to the challenge, as it falls into a tautology: we respond to social facts because we are already shaped by them. We are constrained by social facts into which we are born. It is thus customary to assume that we become aware of social facts only in the case of a crisis. For instance, we feel the pressure of laws when we break them or imagine breaking them. Otherwise, they become mute and invisible.

Instead, I will suggest that psychoanalytical theory can help us break from this vicious circle.[3] Perhaps counterintuitively, psychoanalytical theory shows that the power of a social fact rests not on its taken-for-grantedness but its enigmatic nature; its apparent weakness. We attach ourselves to social facts, not because they are straightforward, definite, and complete, but rather because they are opaque, uncertain, incomplete, and mysterious, or more precisely because of the lack or gap at the heart of social facts. As anthropologist William Mazzarella (2017) writes:

> What attaches us to worlds—to ideologies, to subject positions, to ways of being—is not a watertight and self-sufficient set of propositions that one might accept or reject, believe in or not believe in. Rather, it is, if anything, precisely the opposite. Worlds solicit identification and resonance—and thus also conflict—because of an unresolved lack that gives us a prompt for work, play, and desire. The Indian poet, scholar, and translator A. K. Ramanujan used to say that myths are like crystals: they grow where there's a flaw—in other words, a symptomatic gap that triggers the creative work of imagination and interpretation. (p. 24)

The gap that makes social facts inconsistent is what makes interpellation, our induction into a socio-symbolic world, simultaneously thrilling and unnerving, exciting and paralyzing. Necmi's desire to perform circumcision did not derive from a well-formulated position of Sünnetçi but from the fact that the position was inherently self-contradictory: be a sünnetçi and don't be a sünnetçi. Necmi carved out a space for his desire by embodying the role of Fenni Sünnetçi

(Scientific Circumciser). He imitated itinerant circumcisers without causing a complete breakdown of the boundary between himself and the itinerant circumcisers who were stigmatized in the eyes of medical professionals for (supposedly) having no regard for safety in male circumcision. His relationship with the sünnetçi was, therefore, one of attraction and repulsion that merged admiration with disgust, an ambivalent identification process that secured him a footing in the community.

All attachments and desires are ambivalent in the sense that we are at the same time intractably attached to and defensive against the enigma and pressures of the social world.[4] While stimulated by it, we also anesthetize ourselves to it. Attachment is a force that moves us out of ourselves and "into the world in order to bring closer the satisfying something that [we] cannot generate on [our] own but sense in the wake of a person, a way of life, an object, project, concept, or a scene" (Berlant 2011, p. 1). Yet, simultaneously, we do not bring that "something" too close to ourselves. Thus, balancing himself with Sünnetçi enabled Necmi not to lose himself entirely in the Other—namely, the itinerant circumciser as an abject figure within Turkish nationalist fantasy—the collapse of boundaries that Necmi would have found unacceptable and shameful.

This paradoxical integration of what is simultaneously disavowed, the mixture of binding and unbinding, and the attendant emotions, I suggest, escape the dominant sociological theories of subjectivity, calling for a psychoanalytically informed sociological framework. The following chapters will complement a discursive and institutional analysis of the medicalization of male circumcision in Turkey with an analysis of the changing subjectivities of circumcisers. Close attention will be paid to fantasies that undergird discourses and institutions and that organize and sustain circumcisers' attachments to medicalization even under, and sometimes because of, unfavorable circumstances.[5] Drawing on two years of ethnographic and historical research, I will explore circumcisers' desires to initiate, expand, and implement medicalization in male circumcision as they have traversed major shifts in health care and welfare governance from the 1960s until the present.

Three groups of practitioners have been the major actors in male circumcision: itinerant circumcisers (nonprofessional practitioners), health officers (low-ranking public health workers), and doctors. Their competing desires to not only define who could legitimately perform circumcision but also to alleviate boys' suffering through medicalization have become entangled with developmentalist and neoliberal projects. The main argument of the book is that these practitioners' attachments to the ongoing task of medicalization are structured on *ambivalences* around *ethics of care* and *status*. Accordingly, medical actors confront questions of responsibility, harm, and well-being, as well as problems of status connected to professional boundaries and hierarchies. Regardless of their position in the field of male circumcision—dominant or subordinate, incumbent or challenger, tending to middle-class versus low-income families—ambivalences around care and status emerging from professional domination, market fetishism, and inegalitarian welfare arrangements have been essential to circumcisers' subjectivities.

MALE CIRCUMCISION IN TURKEY

Male circumcision typically refers to the surgical removal of part or all of the penile foreskin. Male circumcision in Muslim-majority Turkey is performed almost universally on young boys for religious, as well as hygienic,[6] reasons and is widely seen as a celebratory rite of passage.[7] The age of circumcision typically ranges from three to eleven, and although neonatal circumcisions have become more common in large cities in recent decades, families tend to have their sons circumcised at an age when they are old enough to remember the event. Often, the boy will wear a circumcision outfit composed of shoes, a cape, a scepter, and a hat (see page xi). Given the absence of an equivalent practice for girls, the rite draws gender as well as religious boundaries, in addition to dividing the male population by age or maturity. Being uncircumcised can be a reason for ridicule and harassment. Contrary to circumcision rites in some other contexts,[8] male circumcision stories in Turkey circulate publicly among adult circumcised men as a homosocial bonding practice.

Given the age range for circumcision and the social value of recollecting the event with or for other men in the future, it is unsurprising that pain is centered in the practice and discourse of male circumcision in Turkey in a way that it would not be if neonatal circumcisions were the norm. Male circumcision is, on the one hand, associated with pain and even punishment: boys may hear cruel jokes about male circumcision, and parents may threaten to call a circumciser and have their sons circumcised if they misbehave, or they might promise them gifts for enduring the operation without showing what would be considered signs of weakness (such as crying). Hospitals and clinics often give boys a "certificate of bravery" or "certificate of manhood" as a testament to their courage and resilience.

On the other hand, families and practitioners have generally viewed circumcision pain as a problem. The widespread preoccupation with circumcision pain encompasses many forms of suffering: pain from cutting off the foreskin, risk of blood loss (which is potentially fatal), long and/or complicated recovery, and trauma. Parents want their sons to have fond memories of their circumcisions, which means minimizing the pain they experience, and they also worry about witnessing their sons' pain themselves. All three groups of practitioners—itinerant circumcisers, health officers, and doctors—have deployed various techniques to manage, if not eliminate, circumcision pain and deliver safe circumcisions. Circumcision pain in Turkey becomes a problem in the interplay of professional and familial values and concerns about well-being and health, both of which intertwine with nationalism, modernization, developmentalism, and neoliberalism.

Male circumcision in Turkey has usually been studied either from public health or a psychodynamics perspective, each approach tending to consider the practice outside of historical and diverse sociopolitical contexts (Cansever 1965; Ozdemir 1997; Ozturk 1973). This book claims that however much the *why* of male circumcision in Turkey has remained constant, suffused with persistent symbolic meanings (birth, male strength, and separation from the mother), the *how* of circumcision has varied across social settings, and the moral, ideological, and practical concerns regarding the performance of circumcision have changed drastically since the early twentieth century. Therefore, male circumcision, I suggest, is neither merely a surgical operation nor a signifier of static "cultures" or "religions" but rather an ever-changing, dynamic, and multifaceted phenomenon embedded within broader institutional and organizational contexts shaped by national and global forces.[9] By offering a bottom-up and historical approach to male circumcision in Turkey, I aim to eschew reifying the practice and instead tie it to such issues as health inequalities, state-building, and market-making—issues that typically fall outside the academic and political discourses on male circumcision in Turkey and elsewhere.

Male circumcision in Turkey represents a curious case of the power of medicine and medicalization in shaping our lives. On the one hand, medicine seems to be omnipresent in the history of Turkey, as it has, from the 1920s onwards, provided language, values, and visions crucial to imagining the nation and healthy population according to modern principles. The power of medicine and medical professionals has extended into new areas, including male circumcision, through health care projects in the more recent developmentalist and neoliberal eras.

On the other hand, the medicalization process has not achieved a complete transformation of male circumcision into a marker of professional prestige, because, as we shall see, a stigma attached to the practice has continued to haunt the medical actors up to the present: the stigma emerging from the fact that male circumcision had been performed by itinerant circumcisers. Moreover, a significant portion of the society, including both practitioners and families, has remained outside the full reach of medicine, including medicalized male circumcision. Asymmetries, exclusion, and inequalities abound. Our analysis of the medicalization of male circumcision will thus attend to the power of medicine as much as its fragility and limits.

STRATIFIED MEDICALIZATION

The medicalization of male circumcision in Turkey has been a stratified process on the sides of both circumcisers and families,[10] and it can be grouped into two waves: *biomedicalization* during the developmentalist era (1960s–1980s) and *psychologization* during the neoliberal era (1980s–present). The two forms of medicalization have gone hand in hand with violent strategies of appropriation, exclusion, and inclusion that transferred control over the practice from itinerant circumcisers to health officers during the developmentalist era and from health officers to doctors during the neoliberal era.

In the 1960s, the Turkish state launched a nationwide developmentalist health care project, inspired partly by the British NHS (National Health Service), to expand public health measures and deliver health care services through state-authorized health care agents (doctors, nurses, midwives, and health officers). The project's goal was to produce healthy and productive citizens according to the medical regime of truth, knowledge, and discourse, via networks of clinics, immunization programs, and childbirth support, to name a few. As part of the project, health officers would marshal professional credentials and legal permission to drive itinerant circumcisers out of practice, gaining control over the jurisdiction of male circumcision while introducing surgical techniques (most notably local anesthesia and sutures), professional skills, and a medical discourse of well-being and health into the practice. Over time, they commodified biomedicalized circumcision and defined circumcision pain as acute, localizable within the body, and caused by organic and physiological dysfunctions. Yet, at the same time, itinerant circumcisers adopted health officers' tools and vocabulary to varying degrees and extended the medicalization of male circumcision as well.

Since the 2000s, the successive AKP (Justice and Development Party) governments have moved away from the developmentalist model in health care and toward a neoliberal model based on principles of efficiency, competition, and consumer choice. The empowerment of a *sovereign consumer* has emerged as a key metric of success in delivering good-quality medical care, and private hospitals have become dominant actors in health care. The neoliberal model has also played itself out in male circumcision as circumcisers have incorporated a biopsychosocial model of harm and care into consumerist comfort and pleasure, not only for boys but also for their families. In doing so, they have legitimized psychic pain, or trauma, as a major concern in male circumcision and commodified the intimacy between families and themselves.

Meanwhile, doctors have in turn delegitimated the expertise and credentials of the previously preferred actors, the health officers, driving them out of the field and replacing them as the new medical authority in male circumcision. While health officers, the winners in the developmentalist era, had also initially adopted a market-oriented professional identity and expanded the second wave of medicalization, they eventually became the losers of the neoliberal period. The gradual shrinkage of those eligible to perform circumcision, from itinerant circumcisers to health officers and then to hospitals, has overlapped with the fusion of circumcision as a commodity with the new ethics of emotional care and harm.

Both waves of medicalization have perpetuated stratification on the level of families as well. Low-income families have remained deprived of what has been considered proper medical care in each era: physical care during developmentalism, and psychological care during neoliberalism. The sons of lower-class families have been circumcised at mass circumcisions, organized at nonmedical settings (such as parks and sports facilities) during the developmentalist era and hospitals during the neoliberal era. In each era, these charity events have taken place at overcrowded venues where practitioners rushed the operations without providing the quality of medical care they provide for the nonpoor. Lack of safe operations has thus been a constant in low-income families' experiences of male circumcision. Practitioners have, in other words, been performing male circumcision within contexts shaped by inequalities.

Alongside each period's reconfigurations of the normative understanding of how male circumcision should be performed, new hierarchies between practitioners have emerged: certain practitioners have been dispossessed in favor of others who have become eligible to perform male circumcision for families of different socioeconomic status. Put differently, the medicalization of male circumcision in Turkey has been patterned over the last century according to both class and professional hierarchies.

Yet, the answer to the question of how actors attach themselves to social structures and experience inequalities, which is essentially a question of how their subjectivities are formed, cannot be gleaned from a structural analysis of stratification that merely focuses on the distribution of goods (medicalized circumcision, in this case). Such a question requires a distinct level of analysis of the mechanisms whereby actors make affective investments in certain positions and relations and not others, as well as of their complex and often contradictory relationships to goods. These investments shape the ways actors act, feel, and organize their practices and are woven into not only the perpetuation of inequalities but also opportunities for social change.

SUBJECTIVITY

The changing subjectivities of drivers of medicalization have received scant attention in the literature on medicalization due to, in part, the ongoing influence of what sociologist Deborah Lupton (1997) calls "the orthodox medicalization critique" (p. 95). According to this critique, which became prevalent from the 1970s onwards, medicalization refers to the immense power amassed by medical professionals, particularly doctors, at the expense of patients and laypeople. This critique condemns medical professionals for their overreaching power, including dictating how people should live their lives, diverting public attention away from socioeconomic problems by rendering them as solely technical issues warranting individual-based solutions, and diminishing people's autonomy in dealing with their own health care (Freidson [1970] 2017; Illich 1976; Szasz 2007; Zola 1972). Professional and economic interests and motives were, it was claimed, transforming such diverse areas and experiences as childbirth, pregnancy, deviance, distress, hyperactivity, menopause, and alcoholism into sites of medical control and regulation, without necessarily proving efficacy in diagnosis and treatment (Conrad 2007; Conrad and Schneider 1980; Scheper-Hughes 1992).

Sociologists, historians, and anthropologists have since used, modified, and expanded the concept of medicalization. They have shown that medicalization, contrary to the assumptions of the orthodox medicalization critique, is less a one-sided imposition than a "multi-dimensional" (Ballard and Elston 2005), contested, negotiated, and ambiguous process whereby laypeople often resist, challenge, and/or reappropriate medicalization to empower themselves (Lock and Kaufert 1998; Nichter 1998). Scholars have also challenged the privileged position accorded by this critique to doctors as the drivers of medicalization, noting that biotech companies, social movements, private insurance companies, and even laypeople can initiate, implement, and demand medicalization in the forms of research, technology, health care infrastructure, health campaigns, and marketing (Bell and Figert 2012; Broom and Woodward 1996; Epstein 1995; Eyal 2013; Clarke 2010; Conrad 2005; Joyce 2008; Hunt 1999; Lewis 1993). These actors have been shown to problematize life, illness, and dying in order to nurture or harness the impulse to prolong biological life (Kaufman 2015; Livne 2019).

However, the link between practitioner subjectivity and medicalization has typically remained outside the scope of both the orthodox medicalization critique and its critical appraisal, with a few exceptions.[11] The orthodox medicalization critique, I suggest, assumes that medicalization is merely a smooth extension of medical professionals' power into new territory. While acknowledging that public desires for medical solutions, products, and technologies are created rather than being given, the critique usually takes for granted medical professionals' own investment in medicalization and its persistence as an innate characteristic of the profession, not as something produced, and thus as unworthy of theoretical and empirical consideration.

In contrast, I will examine the changing subjectivities of circumcisers throughout the medicalization process and show that the relationship between circumcisers and medicalization has been contradictory and ambivalent rather than unequivocal. Close attention will be paid to the pressure of being interpellated as a circumciser while medicalization changes what that means. Circumcisers' ambivalent attachment to the position of circumciser, I will claim, has been a way to make bearable for themselves the "too muchness" (Santner 2001) of recognition—the pressure exerted upon nerves, senses, self-images, and relationships with others.

The pressure associated with the changing signifier of *circumciser* has been structured around two major interrelated concerns: *morality* and *status*. For instance, as discussed in chapter 3, a key component of the medicalization of male circumcision has been the full commodification of biomedicalized male circumcision starting in the 1960s. But circumcisers remained ambivalent toward the image of the profit-seeking circumciser, as communities would frown upon blatant economic motives, which jeopardized circumcisers' status in communities. They thus simultaneously asserted and denied such motives by circumcising boys of low-income families for free. The book traces how such ambivalences act as fragile nodes where circumcisers are integrated into medicalized socio-symbolic worlds.

AMBIVALENCES

Medical sociologists and anthropologists point out ambivalences around morality and status in medical settings.[12] Medical care, they show, comes with anxiety emerging from the experience of attending to, and being held accountable for, others' pain and suffering. Medical professionals often seek to diffuse such anxiety via spatial, temporal, and verbal strategies (Broom, Broom, et al. 2017; Broom, Kirby, et al. 2017; Chambliss 1996; B. Good 1994). For instance, young doctors may overprescribe antibiotics to make sure that their patients will not die under their watch and to defer responsibility to the next treating doctor. Their ambivalence toward caring for others becomes, therefore, a shield against the risk of compromising the image of the good doctor and enables them to tolerate the pressure of being interpellated as doctors (Broom, Broom, et al. 2017).

I contend that dominant sociological theories of subjectivity fail to attend to this ambivalent nature of attachments to subject positions in medical settings (and beyond) and that psychoanalytical theory can redress this problem. A salient approach to subjectivity in medical sociology and anthropology is the interpretivist one closely associated with the philosophy of phenomenology and with social interactionism. To summarize briefly, according to this approach (at the risk of collapsing differences between thinkers such as Schutz, Mead, and Goffman), the act of making sense of the self is simultaneously the act of its constitution. The focus for this tradition is on common, immediate, and lived experiences, as well as the intersubjective realm between social actors and the meaning-making processes whereby social actors anticipate and interpret each other's behavior. Inferences become the fundamental units of analysis, as individuals see themselves in the eyes of others by inferring what others see. We, as "wide-awake" subjects in Schutz's (1967) sense, are bodies endowed with often incomplete practical knowledge of everyday life shaped by commonly held expectations, performances, attitudes, beliefs, and roles—the knowledge that enables us to orient ourselves in routine ways.

The interpretivist approach successfully avoids a deterministic stance concerning the relationship between subjects and society. While we are, it is claimed, constrained by the limitations of language, codes, laws, and norms, we also react to these limitations. Goffman (1990), for instance, argues that we routinely project definitions of situations and work strategically through these presentations to manage ourselves. He makes a distinction between those impressions we "give" and those we "give off": while the former refers to the part of our expressions that we can control and manipulate, the latter refers to the part we have little control over. We operate with incomplete knowledge, and thus our interactions are always fraught with uncertainties—uncertainties that provide the ground for reflection on situations that we find ourselves in. Within this framework, identity becomes an ongoing accomplishment.

From an interpretivist perspective, medicine becomes "a system of symbolic meanings anchored in particular arrangements of social institutions and patterns of interpersonal interactions" (Kleinman 1980, p. 24). The interpretivist approach can help us to analyze the spatial-temporal aspects of not only medical professionals' socialization into their roles but also of illness experiences and clinical encounters from the standpoint of patients (B. Good 1994; Kleinman 1988). By focusing on chronic pain sufferers, for instance, we can attend to the details of patients' meaning-making activities and bodily experiences and how these activities and experiences are interpreted by medical professionals (Buchbinder 2015; M.-J. D. Good 1992). Part of our analytical horizon can be the ways medical actors make sense, or fail to make sense, of their worlds and the conflicts, tensions, and ambiguities that emerge from daily interactions in medical contexts.

Yet, such an approach, I claim, typically fails to account for why and how we become attached to meanings (and norms, roles, and rules). This question never arises because the interpretivist approach assumes that we are fully integrated into the phenomenal world even though our knowledge of it always remains incomplete. What is missing, I suggest, is a robust understanding of humans as not only meaning-making but also desiring beings. Desires emerge mainly because we are never fully integrated into the world. And the psychoanalytical term for this irreducible kernel of subjectivity and attachments is the unconscious.

ATTACHMENTS

For the interpretivist approach, "the unconscious" typically refers to that which evades conscious awareness and yet can be recalled to consciousness at times. However, "the unconscious" in psychoanalysis does not refer to some deep layer of human interiority, as in the latent meanings that are hidden from us (Freud instead calls such meanings "preconscious"). Rather, it should be understood in terms of what Lacan calls "extimacy" (Lacan 1997, p. 139). The unconscious is simultaneously intimate and strange, displacing the binary of interior and exterior. The unconscious permeates the phenomenal world as an absent presence and as a point of breakdown, even as it is also preontological because it points toward that which cannot be assimilated into this world. Sure, the unconscious is always mediated by meaning-making processes in the intersubjective realm, but, and this is crucial, it cannot be reduced to that realm, for it refers to an *excess* of meaning, which thus escapes meaning-centered sociological approaches toward subjectivity.

The unconscious animates our desires and refers to a gap in the phenomenal world that makes the world "fundamentally thrilling and yet unnerving, fascinating and yet overwhelming or revolting" (Fink 1995, p. xii). The unconscious accounts for how and why we are attached to the world in a defensive manner, delicately balancing attraction and repulsion. Identification in psychoanalysis should thus be seen as a double-edged sword. While providing a place in the world, it simultaneously and inevitably carries a traumatic excess: a lurking sense of too-muchness (for instance, having a patient die under your watch) and consequently, the risk of the dissolution of the subject (not being a good doctor). Only through ambivalence can we make recognition bearable for ourselves.

Take the example of humor in medical settings. It is well known that medical professionals use humor to confront the pressure of providing care and of encountering death at hospitals regularly. In an interpretivist approach, we would ask how medical professionals learn to use humor as an implicit and unofficial code through socialization. Humor could be shown to be essential to maintaining an appearance of order in medical settings, and we would gain crucial insights into when professionals use humor, the kinds of humor they use, the significance of medical hierarchies for the use of humor (or lack thereof), and overall, the diverse meanings and functions attributed to humor—meanings and functions embedded within interactions, roles, and status.

However, such an approach would fall short of understanding the contradictory and uncanny nature of humor around life and death in medical settings. Rather, what is needed is an approach that postulates that subjects sustain themselves through unconsciously driven self-sabotage—a fundamental psychoanalytic insight into human subjectivity. Indeed, if medical professionals merely want to avert the displeasure associated with death, why do they still evoke it through humor? Why do they circle around it and not simply avoid it? Paradoxically, humor holds the medical community together, not by avoiding death but by integrating it in a distorted form as an absent presence. Humor thus becomes a mechanism whereby medical professionals attach themselves to their profession by, at the same time, placing safeguards against it, as their profession carries a traumatic excess: encountering death.

The unconscious shapes our desires, which make us, in a way, out of joint with the world in which we are located. It refers to a loaded breaking point that carries the weight of the world. To the extent that it registers the too-muchness of this world, it manifests itself as an excess, an uncanny vitality within the normal and mundane order. Throughout the book, I will be interested in this contradictory and enigmatic aspect of attachments, this uncanny vitality as a mixture of astonishment and uneasiness, which reverberates through utterances, reactions, bodies, and practices—the vitality that shows that although we are not, contrary to what Schutz says, merely wide-awake actors, we nevertheless live in a semi-dream state.

Accordingly, the purpose of the book is to trace how circumcisers have become stimulated by the world, more specifically by the position of the sünnetçi, while anesthetizing themselves to it. In each chapter, I will dramatize ambivalences as constitutive of desires that emerge from different institutional arrangements and discourses about health care, welfare, and male circumcision. In doing so, I will seek to understand how and why circumcisers as agents of medicalization attach themselves to the position of the sünnetçi—whatever the term means in each historical period and context (such as being modern, rational, calculative, self-interested, benevolent, or caring). I will show that circumcisers' ambivalences toward the sünnetçi rest upon the fact that identification with that position carries the potential of transgressing norms, undermining professional ideals, and violating prescriptions such as coming across as too greedy, being mistaken for others, losing (self-)respect, and harming boys, all of which account for the pressure associated with the position of sünnetçi. My argument is that circumcisers have had to circumvent this traumatic excess to enroll themselves in the medicalization process via moral, emotional, and organizational efforts. And these efforts have shaped circumcisers' relationships with themselves and others and have generated pride, anger, shame, guilt, self-doubt, and disgust—a variety of emotions that, the book claims, arise from our ambivalent attachment to the world.

Furthermore, rather than invoking the dualism of subjection versus resistance, a psychoanalytically informed sociological framework can posit ambivalences as the single source of both our tenacious ties to the social order and our capacity to reflect on the same social order in light of the irresolvable quality of such ambivalences—a capacity that may or may not lead to social change. Accordingly, by analyzing the subjectivities of circumcisers I will demonstrate, on the one hand, that they have taken part in reproducing inequalities as relations of dispossession, exclusion, and inclusion—inequalities that are set in motion by state policies and refracted through global market forces. On the other hand, given that the process of subjectivization is unstable and indeterminate, I claim that it always contains the seeds of alternative paths of affective investments that can bloom into new practices. The book will trace such paths as well. For instance, chapter 3 will show how some circumcisers, guilt-ridden for not providing proper care for low-income families' sons, have reorganized mass circumcisions to make them compatible with their moral values.

In recent years, male circumcision has become a controversial topic around the world and to some extent in Turkey. The circumcision debate, I suggest, engages in rather abstract philosophical speculation that limits the ethical and political horizon regarding male circumcision to "for" or "against" options. While the polarized views invoke reified notions such as "rights" (for instance "the right to bodily integrity"), "culture," and "health," I will show that by performing a close analysis of how circumcisers have ambivalently attached themselves to the medicalization process in Turkey, attachments mediated by their interactions with families, it is possible to generate a more nuanced understanding of the various stakes involved in male circumcision and bring forth new questions and elaborations about the ethics and politics of male circumcision.

METHODS

Circumcision and Medicine in Modern Turkey is an ethnographic and historical investigation of the medicalization of male circumcision in Muslim-majority Turkey as it has intersected with state, market, and class-based inequalities over more than a century. It focuses on circumcisers who have introduced new medical models of pain and harm and new standards of care, competed against each other, and served families from different socioeconomic backgrounds. In doing so, I show how they have transformed not only families' medical habitus, but also themselves, and I claim that this transformation has been a fragile, unstable, ambivalent, and anxiety-ridden process wherein being Sünnetçi is persistently rehearsed.

For the research, I conducted interviews with itinerant circumcisers, health officers, and doctors as well as families of varying socioeconomic status and municipal employees involved in organizing mass circumcisions for low-income families. I traveled to twenty-five cities and some of their outlying towns and villages, shaping and reshaping my itinerary to intersect with possible locations my informants reported for itinerant circumcisers. Itinerant circumcisers constituted the only group of practitioners I interviewed who were no longer (or rarely) performing circumcisions, most of whom had carried out their practices without a license, and thus there was almost no contact information available to a nonlocal. I conducted a total of twenty interviews with itinerant circumcisers, almost all in their seventies and eighties. These interviews provided a unique perspective on the past competition between itinerant circumcisers and health officers, a perspective omitted from the dominant narrative that assumes a smooth and conflict-free transition from traditional to scientific circumcision. Health officers were the primary drivers of the medicalization of male circumcision, but itinerant circumcisers, as I demonstrate in chapter 1, also participated in the process and extended the medicalization of circumcision as they tried to sustain their practice against the threat posed by the health officers.

I also interviewed sixty health officers. Health officers are male, state-authorized, licensed, and low-ranked medical professionals (lower than doctors and equivalent to nurses). They typically receive their medical degrees from high school–level or vocational medical schools (sağlık koleji or sağlık meslek lisesi). Most of my interviewees were older than sixty years of age and began to perform circumcision starting in the 1960s as part of the developmentalist health care project. At that time, health officers became eligible to perform what were categorized as minor medical tasks, including circumcision, measuring blood pressure, providing first aid, administering vaccinations, and keeping medical records as well as performing other administrative procedures. Over time, some of them opened their own clinics in cities, but most of them performed circumcisions at families' houses. The Turkish government assigned health officers to various parts of the country, with no plan to inspect them or investigate as to whether they performed male circumcision. As I show in chapter 2, it was mostly left to the discretion of individual health officers whether to begin to perform circumcision, and while many did, some did not.

In addition, I interviewed fifteen doctors (mostly urologists but also general surgeons), senior and young, working at hospitals in three large cities: Istanbul, Izmir, and Ankara. Doctors, although qualified, did not perform circumcision in the past, mainly because they associated the practice with itinerant circumcisers, which in their eyes made the practice irreconcilable with their professional status. Starting in the 2000s, doctors increasingly began to perform circumcision at hospitals, for reasons reflecting the broader imperatives of the consumer-centered neoliberal health care transformation. My interviews with doctors aimed to capture this transition and the differences between their circumcisions and those performed by health officers. These doctors also incorporated and expanded the biopsychosocial model of harm and care in male circumcision.

All of the practitioners I interviewed were male, since women do not typically perform circumcision in Turkey. Throughout the history of the medicalization of male circumcision, performing male circumcision has remained a men's affair, generating economic and symbolic power for men. Being a male researcher not only enabled me to travel around the country alone without much concern for my safety but also allowed me to enjoy a certain level of comfort and easiness in my interactions with the practitioners. Jokes around circumcision and penises, the memory of my own circumcision, and my gender all brought together a set of assumptions, codes, and conventions that facilitated my access to subjects and topics that otherwise would have remained out of reach.[13]

As far as the interviews are concerned, health officers supplied a significant portion of the data, for all of the major transformations in male circumcision in Turkey (biomedicalization, psychologization, developmentalism, and neoliberalism) have taken place during their lifetimes. While itinerant circumcisers eventually embodied a state-based professional identity, namely as Fenni Sünnetçi, and doctors have represented market-oriented professional identity, health officers have embodied both. Following their career trajectories in relation to other practitioners presents a unique window into how these developments have changed the practice and led to inequalities and conflicts.

Moreover, I volunteered at municipalities that organized mass circumcisions for low-income families, helped distribute circumcision outfits to low-income families, and talked with municipality employees of varying ranks. Over time, under the authority of municipalities mass circumcisions have become politicized and, in large cities, channeled toward private hospitals (see chapters 3 and 5). The move toward municipally sponsored mass circumcisions at private urban hospitals has occurred as part of the health care reforms under the AKP—reforms that have increased access to private and public hospitals for low-income families. With the interviews carried out through my volunteering, I aimed to understand how municipalities assess who deserves the aid allocated for male circumcision as well as how and why mass circumcisions are coordinated with private hospitals.

I also attended dozens of individual and mass circumcisions performed by health officers and doctors at homes, clinics, and hospitals in middle-class and working-class neighborhoods. Some practitioners walked me through the operations step by step as they performed them; in some cases, practitioners and families asked me to help them hold boys tight during circumcision. My involvement in these circumcisions was primarily resource-driven: boys under local (not general) anesthesia could, and frequently did, flail, thereby making it difficult for practitioners to perform circumcisions smoothly without causing any harm to the penis. Some parents even asked me to talk to their sons about the operations as their "brother" or "uncle," hoping that I could help to calm them down in the moments before the surgery. At some clinics and mass circumcisions, I joined the audience watching the entertainment staged for boys and families before, during, and after the operations. An underlying concern common to all the circumcisions, however differently they were organized, was the fear surrounding male circumcision shared by boys, practitioners, and families—and the researcher.

My interviews with families about male circumcision proved to be crucial for my project as well. I spoke primarily with parents and grandparents of middle-class and working-class families. These interviews documented the cultural significance of circumcision for families, including those aspects of male circumcision that persist beyond the operation (such as private celebrations) and the generational differences in how circumcision is not only performed but also understood (why, how, and when male circumcision should be done). While my work is centered on circumcisers themselves, my interviews with families enabled me to refine my arguments, since the changes in the practices of circumcisers have been mediated by their interactions with families.

Archival research was essential to this project, especially since the book focuses on historical changes in health care services and male circumcision. I collected newspaper articles, official local and national government documents, and scientific publications on male circumcision from the 1920s to the present. Beyond the knowledge I gained from interviews, these archival materials helped me to grasp the shifts in the cultural significance of male circumcision and in the public discourse on male circumcision: the two waves of medicalization. They also showed how health professionals have framed medicalized male circumcision and sought to reach the wider society. All translations of archival material and interviews in Turkish are mine unless otherwise indicated.

THE OUTLINE

The medicalization of male circumcision in Turkey is a moral, technical, and aesthetic formation wherein circumcisers seek to instill certain medical norms and models of care (biomedical and biopsychosocial models) and induce certain emotions, sensations (such as calmness), and desires (for instance, desires for new medical techniques) in others (boys and their families) via different strategies (for instance, persuasion) used in various media (mass media and face-to-face interactions) for various interrelated purposes (pedagogical, marketing, and therapeutic). Scientific truth, discourse, and knowledge about male circumcision have been entangled with moral rhetoric, professional aspirations, and economic interests. Medicalized male circumcision has been woven into different governmentalities, namely developmentalism and neoliberalism, each making promises, such as for a healthy and productive population and of consumer comfort, respectively—though the promises in both cases have remained unfulfilled for low-income families in each period.

In their attempts to transform families' habitus, circumcisers have transformed themselves as well. Each of the following chapters is organized around different impasses and ambivalences emerging from the dual process in which male circumcision has been medicalized, ambivalences shaping practitioners' state-based and market-oriented subjectivities. These ambivalences have coalesced around status (concern with boundaries and hierarchies) and the ethics of care (centered on themes of responsibility, harm, and well-being) and have been the driving force behind circumcisers' desires for medicalization.

The book is divided into two overarching chronological periods, reflecting the two major healthcare framing categories, developmentalism and neoliberalism, and the two main forms of medicalization: biomedical and biopsychosocial. The chapters within each of the two parts exist in a largely simultaneous time frame, which I investigate from a series of different angles, including different practitioners and different types of circumcisions (individual circumcisions and mass circumcisions).

Chapter 1 analyzes the medicalization of male circumcision from the perspective of itinerant circumcisers. It examines how these circumcisers responded during the developmentalist era to the challenge of health officers encroaching upon their jurisdictional control over the practice. Itinerant circumcisers were trained by apprenticeship, and their skills, knowledge, and techniques were handed down from masters to apprentices, who were often fathers and sons. Although after the 1920s not many of them were legal practitioners, they continued their practice without trouble until the developmentalist era. After the arrival of health officers, itinerant circumcisers could not ignore the medicalization process contradicting and delegitimizing their techniques, knowledge, and skills. To sustain their practices, the chapter argues, itinerant circumcisers mimicked health officers and incorporated surgical techniques to varying degrees while emphasizing their traditional authority.

Chapter 2 examines the reorganization of male circumcision in Turkey under the authority of health officers. Health officers aimed to medicalize the practice of male circumcision and replace itinerant circumcisers by gaining families' support for the new circumcision techniques. The chapter argues that health officers transformed themselves into fenni sünnetçi (scientific circumcisers) through partial imitation of the itinerant circumcisers, known as "sünnetçi" (circumcisers). Fenni Sünnetçi represented a new state-based professional identity essential to reorganizing male circumcision according to biomedical principles in Turkey.

The third chapter examines another status-related dissonance linked with the process of biomedicalization during the developmentalist era: the tension between self-interest as opposed to collective altruism as the orientation normative to the service of others. The arrival of health officers in the 1960s further monetized circumcision services and introduced calculative reasoning in an economic sense into male circumcision. Yet, circumcisers attached themselves to the new position of the calculating self only by distancing themselves from it, since blatant economic self-interest would be denounced by locals. Mass circumcisions organized for low-income families, the chapter claims, thus enabled the practitioners (especially health officers) to sustain their altruistic image ("I am not in this for money. This is a matter of health").

The opening chapter of the book's second part analyzes the neoliberalization of health care services and how this transition transformed the field of male circumcision beginning in the 2000s. It argues that during the neoliberal era circumcisers transformed themselves into *psychologists-by-proxy,* harnessing a trauma-based model of care, pain, and harm to consumerism in middle-class settings. The shift was accomplished by engaging in moral and scientific reflection on what constitutes care and harm in male circumcision, attending to boys' psychology, and creating a *split space* where boys' exposure to each other's fears was minimized, if not eliminated, and hidden from public view. In these settings, circumcisers want to contain boys' fear, not only to prevent it from condensing into trauma but also to eliminate customer dissatisfaction, as emotional distress and outbursts would be seen by families as failures on the part of the circumcisers. In doing so, circumcisers confronted the pressure associated with the demand to produce flawless circumcisions by both avowing and disavowing the inevitable uncertainty and unpredictability inherent in medical care. They attached themselves ambivalently to the position of psychologist-by-proxy.

Chapter 5 returns to the topic of mass circumcisions and analyzes the growing involvement of hospitals in recent decades. Male circumcisions have become a new site of economic capital accumulation for private hospitals, as they have gradually dispossessed health officers of their control over the practice, especially in large cities. As described in chapter 3, some health officers have introduced an appointment system to address deficiencies in the ways mass circumcisions took place during the developmentalist era, such as less than optimal medical care. However, chapter 5 shows how this system has also failed, as mass circumcisions now take place at overcrowded hospital wards, where boys of low-income families are not given proper attention in accordance with what doctors deem good psychological care. The chapter argues that doctors have displaced these failures onto the figures of "Manipulative Child" and "Bad Parents": with the former, they delegitimize boys' psychological suffering and with the latter, they place the blame for this suffering on families. In doing so, they seek to absolve themselves of any responsibility and sustain their professional values. These ideological figures enable them to attach themselves to the position of psychologist-by-proxy by placing a safeguard against it—a safeguard that helps them tolerate the pressure (read: guilt) emanating from performing circumcisions at under-resourced settings.

The conclusion reflects on the relevance of the book's arguments regarding ambivalence to a broader discussion regarding medical care, ethics, and male circumcision. My findings in this study suggest that the global debates over male circumcision need to be revisited, as they either ignore the role of power relations in male circumcision or frame it narrowly according to dichotomies such as autonomy versus coercion or universalism (human rights) versus particularity (cultural relativism). The closing chapter acknowledges that the book

TABLE I: THE ORGANIZATION OF MALE CIRCUMCISION IN TURKEY

	Pre-Developmentalist Period	*Developmentalist Period (1960s–'80s)*	*Neoliberal Period (1980s–)*
Dominant practitioners	Itinerant Circumcisers	Health Officers	Doctors and Hospitals
Types of Medical Model of Pain	——	Biomedical	Biomedical and Psychological

has demonstrated the importance of social and economic motives and interests in medicalizing male circumcision, motives and interests that cannot simply be reduced to a humanitarian ethos. It draws attention to the stratification of the medicalization process and to circumcisers' ambivalent attachments to medicalization in order to suggest that the circumcision debate should extend beyond the simple moral stances of for and against.

When I visited Kırşehir, a mid-sized city in Central Anatolia, my goal was to talk to Abdals—a group of itinerant circumcisers known also for their musical activities nationally and internationally. The renowned Abdal musician and folk music singer Neşet Ertaş was born in this city. He played and sang at local weddings in Kırşehir, though he never performed circumcision. He rose to fame in the 1970s and '80s when he was singing folk songs (türkü) for the national public broadcaster (TRT), a state-owned national network. TRT has routinely aired other Abdal musicians' concerts as well, a clear testament to Abdal musicians' place in the nation's cultural scene. Yet, their circumcision activities have never received such publicity.

To reach the Abdals, I contacted Mustafa, the head of a cultural center that in 2011 launched a cultural heritage project about Kırşehir's history. The project promoted the city's artistic, religious, architectural, and archeological heritage, including the Abdals' musical talents. After he provided an overview of their ongoing project, I asked him whether the project had considered including Abdals' circumcision activities as well. Baffled by my question, he responded: "we never thought about talking to Abdals about circumcision . . . Maybe we should." He offered to put me in touch with an itinerant circumciser. He and I then went to the nearby village of Sünnetçi Kamil, an eighty-one-year-old itinerant circumciser.

Sünnetçi Kamil, well known in the city both as an Abdal musician and a circumciser, had decided to quit circumcision in the 1990s when the Turkish Ministry of Culture and Tourism employed him as a musician. Mustafa, Sünnetçi Kamil, and I sat down on stools in front of Sünnetçi Kamil's mud-brick house, and as Mustafa introduced us to each other, I asked Sünnetçi Kamil's permission to interview him about male circumcision. He also seemed to be taken aback by my interest:

> Look, they did all the research about culture, Abdal traditions, and music. Even foreign researchers came and talked to me. They all asked me about

the musical instruments that I was playing. But circumcision . . . It is the
first time someone wants to talk to me about circumcision.

As the next chapter explains in detail, starting in the early twentieth century
Turkish elites considered male circumcision part of the Turkish "culture" insofar as this religious practice came under medical authority—an approach
consistent with the official Turkish nationalism's pragmatic mobilization of
Islam in imagining, creating, and sustaining social cohesion while staking
claims to the modern and secular world. Accordingly, the new symbolic status
of male circumcision was disseminated via various media, such as circumcision celebration photos representing Turkey as an exotic touristic destination
with religious motifs. However, itinerant circumcisers like Sünnetçi Kamil
have been absent from this secular and nationalist repertoire of memories,
images, and symbols—a repertoire arranged to be a source of pride and honor.
Hence Kamil's surprise about my interest in his circumcision practices.

This chapter examines two interrelated processes from the perspective of itinerant circumcisers: the medicalization of male circumcision and
the obliteration of itinerant circumcisers from the national scene. Although the
Turkish state in 1928 excluded itinerant circumcisers (also known colloquially
as "alaylı"[1]), these circumcisers continued performing circumcision without
much trouble in the early decades of the Republic. That said, with the growing
number of health officers starting in the 1960s, itinerant circumcisers faced a
dilemma. On the one hand, they wanted to sustain their practice for economic
and symbolic reasons. On the other hand, they could no longer ignore the
medicalization process initiated by health officers—a development delegitimizing itinerant circumcisers' long-standing and well-entrenched authority
among rural communities as well as the techniques, knowledge, and skills be-
queathed from generation to generation. To manage this dilemma, this chapter argues, itinerant circumcisers attached themselves to the medicalization
process *ambivalently*: they mimicked health officers while also invoking their
traditional authority backed by communal recognition, an appeal that served
as a safeguard against the threat of medicalization. They bound themselves,
paradoxically and partially, to what otherwise destabilized their legitimacy.

In what follows, I first describe different groups of itinerant circumcisers,
their training of apprentices, and the socio-symbolic structures in which their
circumcision activities were located. Then, I examine how the medicalization of the 1960s transformed their practices and subjectivities as they were
challenged by health officers. In partially imitating health officers, itinerant
circumcisers (most of whom were performing circumcision without a license)
wanted as much to maintain their practices in a context increasingly shaped

by competition with health officers as to adopt the emerging medical ethos of well-being, safety, and health around male circumcision. This subjective transformation represented a response to both moral and status-related dissonances, reanimating itinerant circumcisers' desires to continue performing circumcision under increasingly unfavorable conditions.

PRE-MEDICALIZATION

The circumcision field in the pre-medicalization period was fragmented, as there was no unifying authority that would oversee itinerant circumcisers' activities and connect them according to a certain shared set of rules, procedures, and codes. Nor, contrary to the Turkish modern and nationalist discourse's sweeping generalization, did itinerant circumcisers constitute a homogenous group. Itinerant circumcisers differed from each other in terms of ethnic and religious backgrounds, the regions where they worked, and other occupations they held. In our analysis of itinerant circumcisers, we must take into account such social and cultural differences, as they shape how itinerant circumcisers are known, perceived, and treated by families and other circumcisers.

One group of itinerant circumcisers I interviewed was the Abdals. Besides performing circumcision, Abdals played musical instruments and sang at weddings over summers, and both income-generating activities were carried out solely by men living an itinerant life across generations. As I explain in more detail later, their musical skills were, as in male circumcision, transmitted through apprenticeship, usually from fathers to sons. Among their most common instruments were clarinet, shrill pipe, cümbüş (a traditional Turkish instrument with twelve strings and no frets, resembling a banjo), and darbuka (a goblet-shaped hand drum). However, Abdals have fallen out of fashion over the last decades due to the growing consumer demand for wedding halls, which typically offer live bands as part of their standard packages.

Furthermore, ethno-religious discrimination on a daily basis has exacerbated Abdals' economic challenges. The Turkish public often compares Abdals to other stigmatized groups such as the Romani people, alluding to their shared itinerant lifestyle. Another layer of exclusion and vulnerability comes from their religious identity: most Abdals are Alevis—a religious minority in Turkey. The Turkish state sought to control religion by positing Sunnism, the largest branch of Islam, as the true Islam and a social glue that binds people together. This sectarian position not only manifested in discriminatory policies concerning religion (for instance, refusing to officially recognize the "cemevi," the Alevis' place of worship) but also contributed to ordinary and mass forms of violence that state and non-state actors perpetrated against Alevis

(Karakaya-Stump 2020, 2018). The stigma attached to Alevi Abdals accounts in part for my interviewees' difficulty in finding jobs in public or private sectors.

Another group of circumcisers I talked to was the Tillolulars (circumcisers from Tillo). Tillo is a district of Siirt, a city located in southeastern Turkey. The name of Tillo, known as "the center of the holy ones," is derived from the Arabic *Tall*, meaning "hill, elevation." As part of Turkification policies requiring that the names of cities, towns, and villages be derived from Turkish words, the name of Tillo was changed to Aydınlar in 1964 and remained so until the then prime minister Recep Tayyip Erdoğan changed it back again to its original name, Tillo, in 2013—another of Erdoğan's ideological maneuvers to revive the (so-called) glorious days of the Ottoman Empire. Due to having an itinerant lifestyle, the Tillolulars were also called "wanderers" by locals in the region.

Up until the 1980s, male circumcision, unlike for Abdals and barbers, was the sole source of livelihood for many adult men in Tillo. Circumcisers from Tillo, also trained by apprenticeship, traveled to Iraq and Syria as well as the eastern and southeastern parts of Turkey for circumcision. Over the last three decades, a flow of migration has occurred from Siirt to larger cities such as Istanbul, Ankara, and Van due to the shrinkage of available jobs, the escalating war between PKK (Kurdistan Workers' Party) and the Turkish army in the 1990s, and the Iraq War in the 2000s. The wars considerably limited the geographical scope of the Tillolulars' activities around the region, too. As a result, the number of circumcisers from Tillo has decreased over time.

The third group of circumcisers I interviewed was barbers. Traditionally, young barbers first assisted their masters, the same masters from whom they learned the skill of barbering, as apprentices during circumcisions and then began to perform circumcision on their own. My research also showed that barbers until the early twentieth century were seen as doctors in some parts of Turkey (for instance, Adıyaman) as some, besides circumcising boys and working as a barber, also extracted teeth without anesthesia.

Some of my interviewees did not belong to any of these groups, and all the itinerant circumcisers, except for those from Tillo, engaged in other trades and businesses as well: some were barbers, musicians, carpenters, or farmers, and others owned small shops. Itinerant circumcisers sometimes distinguished themselves from each other to stress their uniqueness and superiority over each other. More specifically, the stigma attached to Abdals informed how other circumcisers perceived their circumcision activities. When I asked circumcisers from Tillo whether, besides performing circumcision, they played music at circumcision events, some of them got upset: "No, we are not Abdals! We only perform circumcision." To assert their difference from other itinerant circumcisers relying on non-circumcision activities for income as well, they prided themselves on being descendants of saints from Tillo and regarded performing circumcision—their sole job—as a pious activity. In the same vein, when I asked barbers about their daily travels for circumcision, my question bothered some of them, as they too felt as though I was comparing them to Abdals.

Itinerant circumcisers performed circumcision in distinct territories partitioned according to networks established over time and tried not to encroach on each other's territory. Engaging in other trades helped some itinerant circumcisers broaden their client base for circumcision without causing territorial conflicts with others. For instance, locals knew Abdals first and foremost as musicians since they went to weddings in villages, an advantage that boosted their reputation as circumcisers as well. Similarly, having regular customers for haircutting at their barbershops endowed barbers with visibility and connections that proved to be useful for their circumcision activities too. I asked Sünnetçi Selim, a barber and a circumciser, about his jobs:

AUTHOR: Did being a barber give you an advantage in circumcision?
SELİM: Yes. I already knew how to use a straight razor. My master taught me. He made me work on a balloon. He put shaving cream on it and I gently shaved it off.
AUTHOR: What about clients? Did it help you meet people, too?
SELİM: Of course. No one would trust me if I were not a barber. It is important to be a tradesman [esnaf]. They trusted my skills. They were my regular customers at my barbershop.
AUTHOR: Did they call you "barber" or "circumciser?"
SELİM: First, barber. Then, they saw that I did circumcisions too and started calling me "circumciser." At some point, they even called me "doctor" [he smiles]. But then health officers came along. It is good that they did, but not all of them were good circumcisers.
AUTHOR: Why not?
SELİM: They did not know how to cut. They made penises look ugly.

Working on a balloon was a common training practice among barbers, as it helped maintain attention, develop precision and control, and complete the task with care, the same qualities required for safe male circumcision. And besides versatile skills, barbering also provided Selim with social capital based on trust, which he could transfer to his circumcision practice.

As health officers initiated the medicalization process in the 1960s, all itinerant circumcisers gradually adopted medical expertise to varying degrees. To better understand the circumstances of this transformation, the next section takes a closer look at the patriarchal relations in which itinerant circumcisers lived and performed circumcision. It illuminates the importance of male circumcision as a source of economic and symbolic power for men and boys, whose status was organized by gender- and age-based hierarchies and domination.

CLASSIC PATRIARCHY AND APPRENTICESHIP

In summer 2014 I visited a small northern city of Turkey that I had never been to before. My goal was to find itinerant circumcisers for an interview, and as usual I went straight to a coffeehouse (kahvehane) at the city center. Dating as far back as the Ottoman Empire, coffeehouses in Turkey have been important public places where adult men meet, drink coffee or tea, play games, smoke tobacco, and exchange news (Kırlı 2004). Especially in small cities, towns, and villages, coffeehouses play a crucial role in forging personal connections and networks, and my gender identity, despite being a stranger, enabled me to use coffeehouses as a point of contact for my research.

As I walked into the coffeehouse, I introduced myself to the çaycı (waiter) and asked him if he knew any circumcisers in the area. He asked around, and a customer referred me to an itinerant circumciser, Mehmet. I greeted Mehmet and explained my research to him. He agreed to talk to me, but with one condition: I could neither take notes nor record the interview. His request was not unusual; few of the itinerant circumcisers, almost none of whom were in practice at the time of the research, permitted me to record the interviews, though some let me write down notes. Their cautious stance stemmed from the fact that, with a few exceptions, all had circumcised boys without a license for decades.

With my assurance regarding confidentiality and anonymity, Mehmet pulled up a chair for me, and we sat down for the interview. As I was elaborating on my research goal, we took a break, since Mehmet had to attend the daily prayer service at a nearby mosque. Once he was back, I could now, he said, take notes, but I still could not use my recorder. Having had established rapport with him, I wanted to know more about his training as a young apprentice.

Mehmet started shadowing his father during circumcisions at the age of eight. Together, they walked from one village to another during the summers for circumcision, announcing their arrival in a village with a shout, and had boys gather at village centers for circumcision or circumcised them at their homes. During the travels, Mehmet held various responsibilities. He carried his father's toolkit, which helped him gain familiarity with the instruments. He also helped his father circumcise boys efficiently and safely by holding them: he placed boys younger than him in his lap, put their arms inside and looped around their legs, and kept the legs as wide and tight as possible so that the boys would not fidget from fear or pain and injure themselves or circumcisers.[2]

As for circumcisions for boys older than Mehmet, senior elders (such as their fathers or uncles) held the boys while Mehmet stood near his father, handing him the tools as needed. As part of his training, he also practiced and improved his cutting skills on a sheep's small intestines with a straight razor. His father highlighted to him the importance of precision, focus, and dexterity. "Then, I started performing circumcision on my own," he said. A hint of discontent in his voice made me curious:

AUTHOR: Did you want to do this job?
MEHMET: Not really. My dad forced me. He said, "I will never forgive you if you don't do it" [hakkımı helal etmem sana]. My grandfather was also a circumciser during the Ottoman era. But I did not want to do it.
AUTHOR: Why not?
MEHMET: It is too stressful. What if it bleeds too much? I could not make much money, either. Other circumcisers did.
AUTHOR: Oh really?
MEHMET: Yes. I think because of the area where I worked. Other areas were better.
AUTHOR: How did your first circumcision go?
MEHMET: There were göçerler [nomadic people] living in tents. My dad did not know about it [his first circumcision]. He was supposed to circumcise them but could not make it. I told them that I could do it instead and eventually did it. I was fifteen years old at that time and the kid I circumcised was older than me.

His father's insistence that Mehmet continue a family tradition should be situated within what feminist scholar Deniz Kandiyoti (1988) calls "classic patriarchy." In the pre-1950s, eighty percent of the population was living in rural areas in Turkey, and classic patriarchy, a form of patriarchy that also existed in other parts of the Muslim Middle East,[3] as well as in South and East Asia, was the dominant social system for allocating material and symbolic resources (such as land and honor). In classic patriarchy, three generations typically cohabit, and their living arrangement is structured around age-based deference and distinct yet interrelated male and female hierarchies. Classic patriarchy appropriates women's labor and their reproductive capacities via mechanisms of patrilineage. Women's life chances are limited to their roles in family and marriage: their social mobility depends on their ability to produce male offspring who can continue the male lineage. Newlywed women submit themselves to the male authority, hope to have a son, and eventually, as senior women, control the domestic labor of their daughters-in-law.[4]

Another characteristic of male dominance in classic patriarchy is the honor code, which regulates female sexuality according to the norms of purity and chastity. Via this code, classic patriarchy (and other forms of patriarchy today) shapes and limits not only women's life chances but also their physical mobility. Wandering was a male privilege, as women's public presence and their interactions with other men were (and often still are, to varying degrees) under strict male scrutiny.[5] Given the itinerant lifestyle that performing circumcision entailed, the moral disciplining of women and girls in public can be seen as another ground for their exclusion from the socially valued position of Sünnetçi among locals.

In classic patriarchy, productive and reproductive activities are not gendered in a clear-cut fashion: women, to a considerable degree, participate in production, and men have some responsibilities in reproduction, especially that of male labor (as in the case of male circumcision) (Özbay 1995). Young sons, when married, could make claims over resources (for instance, land and the position of master in male circumcision) and extract themselves from the hierarchical relationship with their fathers. In male circumcision, sons' subordination to fathers during training was essential to transmitting skills, knowledge, and prestige from one generation to another. Once they completed their training, apprentices moved to the next step: performing circumcision on their own. The transition to mastership was devoid of any concomitant ceremonial or institutionalized recognition, yet it still required masters' evaluation of their apprentices' skills and competence. There were, however, exceptions like Mehmet (described above) and Barber Hasan.

Barber Hasan, a seventy-seven-year-old itinerant circumciser, performed his first circumcision in 1963 at the age of twenty-seven. He was born and grew up in Malatya, an eastern city of Turkey, where he could complete only primary school since his family lacked the financial means for further studies. Instead, his father sent him to a barber as an apprentice to learn what Hasan called the "art." Besides working as a barber, Hasan's master performed circumcision, and he brought Hasan along. After careful and consistent observation and then helping his master, Barber Hasan one day decided to circumcise a boy on his own:

AUTHOR: What was your first circumcision like?

BARBER HASAN: One day, I was at this village and the locals asked for my master, but they could not reach out to him. I said, "I can also do it." They were surprised: "Do you know how to circumcise?" I said, "Yes." I lied, of course. Then, I went to the house where the children were waiting for circumcision. In those times, we used to place the child on the kirve's lap and pull the curtain so that nobody would see us.[6] Anyways, I asked them to pull the curtain. If I started shaking, I did not want people to see it. Then, they pulled the curtain. I cut them off. I stayed in the village for four or five days. I could not go back home. I wanted to make sure that the kids were okay. Then, I came back home, and now I was a circumciser.

Barber Hasan's worry concerning his performance as a circumciser was intense but not unusual. The health officers and itinerant circumcisers I spoke with often highlighted the experiences of stress and anxiety occasioned by uncertainties around the operation, especially when they first began to perform circumcision. The possibility of causing harm to boys was sometimes so overwhelming that they couldn't sleep later that night, or some even visited families in the middle of the night to check on boys. The additional intensity of Barber Hasan's anxiety came from the fact that he performed his first circumcision without his master's permission.

Apart from rare cases like Barber Hasan and Mehmet, individual masters typically decided when their apprentices should start circumcising boys without their supervision. Haydar, an eighty-two-year-old circumciser from a Central Anatolian city, began to perform circumcision at the age of twenty and retired after his heart attack twenty years ago. His family (his wife, his sons, and his daughters-in-law) joined us for the interview as well:

AUTHOR: Did you always use a straight razor?

HAYDAR: Yes, I was using a new one for each circumcision. It was cleaner that way.

AUTHOR: And how did you learn it?

HAYDAR: My father taught me. He is now dead. I observed his hand, his foot, his cutting, the way he held his straight razor, and the way he was laying out the instruments. My master was my father. He is no longer alive.

AUTHOR: Who taught your father?

HAYDAR: I think his father taught him. I am not sure. I learned it from him. We went to villages together. People knew us.

AUTHOR: So were you traveling around with your father?

HAYDAR: Yes, my father was doing the cutting. I watched him: how he held the spindle, cut it off, prayed, and then dressed it [the incision].

AUTHOR: How many kids did you and your father circumcise together each day?

HAYDAR: It depends. Three kids from one village, five kids from another. Some days we traveled around all day but did not perform any circumcision. But when we did it, it was more than one kid. People knew us. When we arrived at a village, people would say, "Here are our circumcisers."

AUTHOR: How did you travel around?

HAYDAR: On foot and sometimes by car. We used to stay over in a village. Since they knew us, they would have us at their places overnight.

AUTHOR: How did you decide to perform circumcision yourself?

HAYDAR: My father watched me circumcise a couple of kids and said I was ready. May Allah not let me make a mistake.

AUTHOR: I see. How did your first circumcision go?

HAYDAR: I was nervous. But I got used to it over time.

Young apprentices like Sünnetçi Haydar, through their training, acquired a "feeling for the game" (Bourdieu and Wacquant 1992, 128) by carefully watching their masters' styles, skills, and instruments at different stages of the operation. Masters became a "visual model" (Wacquant 2004, p. 113) for apprentices, who occupied various positions as they were holding boys tightly or handing their masters circumcision instruments. Masters then observed their apprentices' circumcisions, provided feedback, tracked their progress, and finally, like Haydar's father, allowed their apprentices to continue performing circumcision independently. The cycle, at least in principle, continued when the new masters trained their own sons.

At the heart of apprenticeship lies reciprocal generosity between masters and apprentices, which involves an exchange of time, knowledge, labor, and skills. This type of reciprocal generosity can be overshadowed by masters' anxiety about controlling the flow of knowledge, techniques, and skills—an anxiety that can at times even deter masters from teaching their crafts for fear of future competition. In the case of Cretan male artisans in Greece, for instance, as shown by the anthropologist Michael Herzfeld (2004), apprentices have learned despite their masters' ambivalent attitudes toward their apprentices. For these artisans, the acquisition of knowledge becomes coupled with discouragement that is both "the instrument and object of the apprentices' socialization" (p. 63).

In contrast to Cretan male artisans who employ apprentices outside the kinship network, the master-apprentice relationships among itinerant circumcisers in Turkey, except for some barbers, remained within the father-son bond. Some itinerant circumcisers refrained from sharing their recipes of herbs with other circumcisers and often refused to train strangers. Performing circumcision was a source of (gendered) symbolic and economic power for itinerant circumcisers, and classic patriarchy ensured the transference of this status as well as the associated knowledge, techniques, and skills over successive generations of the same descent line.

However, as promising as performing circumcision was, some itinerant circumcisers initially had ambivalent feelings concerning the occupation, and unlike Mehmet, not every son of itinerant circumcisers eventually chose their father's path. One reason for their reluctance was their worry about getting caught by state authorities, as they knew they could not get a license. The other reason was the anxiety around the harm that circumcision could cause in children. For instance, for years Mesut traveled with his father to villages and assisted him with circumcisions, but he never started his practice. When I interviewed his father, Mesut also joined us:

AUTHOR: Why didn't you want to perform circumcision?
MESUT: It is too dangerous. It can bleed. I used to run away when my father was about to cut it off [he smiles]. My father forced me to do it, but I was too afraid to use a straight razor on children. What if you cut the whole thing off? I was telling my father not to do it because it is too dangerous. None of my brothers did it, for the same reason. If you did something wrong, you can ruin the kid's life. He can't get married and have kids.

For Mesut, the risks involved in male circumcision felt like too much to bear, as it generated anxiety around harm and care, thus discouraging him from performing circumcision. This was also true for other senior itinerant circumcisers' sons, many of whom pursued other lines of work or business such as those of factory workers or shopkeepers. Juxtaposing these men's relative autonomy over their future with Mehmet's acquiescence to his father's wishes suggests that the relation of dependence between sons and fathers in classic patriarchy was flexible rather than rigid.

The Turkish state's intervention in male circumcision in 1928 should be seen as an attempt to replace the classic patriarchy's system of organizing the reproduction of circumcisers along patrilineal lines with modern educational institutions that not only medicalized the practice but also assumed control over who could and could not access the medicalized expertise (techniques, knowledge, and skills). The section on circumcision in the 1928 law prohibited circumcisers without license and medical education from performing circumcision. And while the prohibition did not apply to female health professionals, women were excluded from the field by the gendered structure of medical education combined with deep-seated cultural beliefs and perceptions about the necessity of circumcisers being men. Performing male circumcision remained a man's affair, which is still the case today. As a consequence, the law inadvertently set the stage for the jurisdictional struggles that would take place between the two groups of male practitioners: health officers and itinerant circumcisers.

How did the medicalization of male circumcision during the developmentalist era affect itinerant circumcisers' practices? How did itinerant circumcisers with no role in the state-led project of the socialization of health care services experience and respond to health officers' intrusion into their territory? How did itinerant circumcisers seek to protect their authority and maintain their practice in a context where the meanings of circumcision and Sünnetçi were drastically changing?

DISPOSSESSION

The 1928 law prohibited itinerant circumcisers (as unlicensed practitioners) from continuing their practice and threatened them with punishment. As I discuss in detail in the next chapter, the main rationale behind the state intervention was that itinerant circumcisers were viewed as a threat to the health of boys. With this law, the Turkish ruling elites deployed what sociologist Mara Loveman (2005) calls a "strategy of usurpation": a strategy whereby a modern state extends its legitimacy by stripping non-state actors of "the means and/or authority to continue their traditional practices and taking over these practices themselves, imbuing them with new meanings in the process" (p. 1661). This strategy laid the groundwork for coordinating the practice of male circumcision under medical authority by stipulating that a license granted by public authorities and medical credentials be the prerequisite for performing circumcision. In strict legal terms, the itinerant circumcisers without medical training or license became illegitimate. Thus, some itinerant circumcisers had to pay a fine or even got arrested.

However, there was an exception to the law: the 58th and 59th clauses stated that circumcisers with at least ten years of experience could receive a special permit (sünnetçi ruhsatnamesi) from the Ministry of Health and Social Assistance. Moreover, circumcisers who did not meet the ten-year threshold could still receive the same license on the condition that they observed operations performed by a specialist in a hospital for two to six months and passed the qualification exams.

Two of the itinerant circumcisers I interviewed managed to get short-term licenses in the 1970s (both refrained from disclosing the expiration dates). Sünnetçi Sinan applied to a state hospital in his district and received basic training for six months. "They taught me to use local anesthesia and suture," he said. He then performed a few procedures under the supervision of doctors and got his license. The other itinerant circumciser was Kamil, the Abdal musician introduced at the beginning of the chapter. He wanted a license for peace of mind:

Health officers were giving me a hard time for not having a license. So, I applied to the health board to get one and they sent me to a nearby hospital.

On that day some boys were going to be circumcised at the hospital, and the doctors asked me to circumcise them. As I told you before, I did my military service as a sergeant in the public health department [Sıhhiye]. I already knew how to dress a wound and give an injection. They gave me a certificate that allowed me to dress wounds, give an injection, and perform circumcision. I always kept it in my tool bag so that no one could interfere with my business and I would not be worried.

The license was, Sünnetçi Kamil said, just a piece of paper and didn't mean anything beyond offering a safeguard against health officers. He emphasized that he had already been confident in his skills before receiving the license—the skills he inherited from his ancestors and learned during the military service.

However, most itinerant circumcisers could not benefit from this exemption. And while itinerant circumcisers' encounters with the force of the law during the early decades of the twentieth century remained sporadic, as the Turkish state had not yet assumed a major role in public health, the health care project of the 1960s, which was the largest health care project in the nation's history, changed this situation: the number of health officers who began to challenge itinerant circumcisers increased significantly, and at the same time, security forces tightened control over itinerant circumcisers. Thus, for example, Mehmet (who, contrary to his wishes, eventually started his own practice) faced problems:

AUTHOR: Did your father get into trouble with authorities?

MEHMET: No, because he attended a training [kurs] at a hospital. He performed a couple of circumcisions there and got a license saying "he can perform circumcision." I also tried to get a license. I even went to Ankara [the capital of Turkey], but they favored health officers. They did not give it to me. There were more health officers by then, anyway.

AUTHOR: Did you get into trouble with authorities because of this?

MEHMET: Yes, I did. A health officer reported me and I stood before the court. They sentenced me to fifteen days of jail. But since that was my first strike, they let me go on the condition that I would not continue doing it. I did, of course.

AUTHOR: What exactly happened at the court?

MEHMET: I was honest. I told the judge that I indeed performed circumcision and learned it from my father, who was well known here. It turned out that I had even circumcised the prosecutor's son! They asked, "So, you did not have a license?" I said, "No." Then, he said, "But I saw how you did it. You did it well."

AUTHOR: What happened after that? Did you get into any trouble again?

MEHMET: Of course I did. Normally, they clear your record after five years. But in the meantime, they [health officers] reported me a few more times. But I continued performing circumcision. I had been doing it for years by then.

The Turkish state's health care project accounts for the different treatments that Mehmet and his father received from the state authorities. By the time Mehmet came of age and began to perform circumcision on his own, his area saw an upsurge in the number of health officers who wanted to take over the practice. Mehmet had been a well-known circumciser in his small city, as attested ironically by the fact that he had circumcised the son of the person who prosecuted him. That said, a variety of state actors—health officers, the local health care department at which Mehmet applied for a license, and the court—came into alignment to dispossess Sünnetçi Mehmet of his economic and symbolic power: his income and prestige.

The same alignment of the 1960s was gaining momentum in other areas of Turkey as well. Sünnetçi Selim, a seventy-five-year-old man, was another itinerant circumciser who was denied the special permit. I talked to him in a village in western Turkey. Like Mehmet, he did not let me use my recorder for the interview and asked suspiciously if I was working for a newspaper. Once I assured him that I was not a journalist and would use a pseudonym, we sat down for the interview on his porch and talked about his encounters with state authorities:

SELİM: I was once brought to the court.

AUTHOR: Who reported you?

SELİM: A health officer. He was older than me. He told the court that I did not have a license. He then died.

AUTHOR: When was this?

SELİM: Sometime between 1965 and 1970.

AUTHOR: Why did he do that?

SELİM: I corrected his operations. He had circumcised five or six boys, had cut off very little, and then had left them like that. I finished the rest of it. He saw me as a rival.

AUTHOR: And he heard of this and took you to the court?

SELİM: Yes.

AUTHOR: What happened, then? How did it get resolved?

SELİM: The judge said, "Don't do it if you don't have a license." They gave me a warning. But I continued. I said, "What license? I inherited this from my ancestors."

AUTHOR: Did you ever try to get a license?

SELİM: I did. But since I am not okullu [formally educated], they did not give it to me. Maybe, if I knew someone in Ankara, I could get it.

By mentioning Ankara, the capital of Turkey and the center of the Turkish government, Sünnetçi Selim alluded to nepotism as a common way of circumventing the bureaucratic rules and regulations for personal gain in Turkey—a form of nepotism that typically relies on affiliations and loyalties around kinship, political party, and town or city of origin, none of which applied to Sünnetçi Selim. And neither the traditional authority he invoked ("I inherited this from my ancestors") nor his style and skills were considered valuable by the state authorities. In contrast, Selim believed that his style and skills made his circumcisions' aesthetics superior to those performed by the senior rival who reported him. He even added humorously: "I make the penis look like a candy apple." Yet, these qualities fell short of giving him a competitive advantage against his rival, whose legitimacy was backed by the law.

The emerging state-centered network around male circumcision at times involved security forces, as well. Examining the cultural aspects of state formation, scholars have expanded upon Weber's (1946) definition of the state as a "human community that (successfully) claims the monopoly of the legitimate use of violence within a given territory" (p. 78).[7] By emphasizing the contingent nature of legitimacy, they argue that state monopoly of violence is neither a given nor a finished product but rather must be produced, reasserted, and justified—a process susceptible to contestation and conflicts. The state's monopoly over violence, in other words, works to the fullest only when violence remains in the background of social relations as a threat. Resorting to actual violence would reveal weakness, rather than strength, on the part of the state that relies on citizens' consent for its policies. Some itinerant circumcisers encountered state violence of this kind.

I talked to Cemal, a sixty-five-year-old itinerant circumciser and an Abdal musician, in a small village in the central Anatolian region. Sünnetçi Cemal began to circumcise boys right after he got married in 1967 and circumcised his sons and grandsons too. He had learned to perform circumcision from his uncle:

CEMAL: I played musical instruments at weddings until I got married. We learned the repertoire through oral transmission [kulaktan dolma]. We are not schooled. After I got married, I started performing circumcision and did it for forty-five years.

When I asked him about his interactions with health officers, he responded:

CEMAL: There was a health officer who watched me perform circumcision. He said, "You are a master. You should teach me." Allah is the Witness; I did not help him [smiles]. I was making a living from this. That's why I did not teach him.

AUTHOR: Did you ever get into trouble with authorities?

CEMAL: The gendarmerie came to the village.[8] They wanted me to bring the instruments to the police station. They said, "You don't have a license." What license? [he raises his voice] I inherited this craft from my ancestors. What are you talking about? Then a well-respected elder in our village confronted them, and I did not have to go to the police station. They left me alone but arrested another circumciser because the kid he circumcised died.

AUTHOR: When did this happen? Did you get into trouble again?

CEMAL: After the 1980s. Yes, I got into trouble again but continued to perform circumcision.

Sünnetçi Cemal, worried about potential future competition, declined to train the young and inexperienced health officer. Yet, as an unlicensed practitioner, he faced another threat to his practice when the gendarmerie attempted to interfere with his circumcision. The locals knew both his father and his grandfather, who also served the same village. Thus, his recourse to traditional authority backed by the communal support he had built over the years helped him escape the gendarmerie's intervention and continue his practice until he retired.

Bülent, a sixty-three-year-old sünnetçi, had a hostile interaction with the gendarmerie, too. I talked to him in a small village in a small-sized central Anatolian city. Sünnetçi Bülent learned the craft from his father and had been circumcising boys independently since the age of twenty. At the time, he was training his youngest son as well, but he doubted his son's plans: "I don't think he will do it because he might not want to get into trouble." As an unlicensed practitioner himself, Sünnetçi Bülent's insights about his son were informed by his own experience:

AUTHOR: Did you have any problem with health officers?

BÜLENT: Not much. Once I was circumcising a kid and a health officer was present, too. He said to me, "You should not do this. What if it bleeds?" The boy's father replied, "It is none of your business. The child is mine. If it bleeds, it will be my child who would bleed."

AUTHOR: What about the gendarmerie?

BÜLENT: One day, I was going to perform a circumcision in [X] village. A soldier came and said, "You do not have a permit. You can't do it." But the family had known me for years. The child's father scolded him, saying, "It is none of your business. The child is mine." The soldier walked up to the sergeant, who instructed him to let me complete the circumcision and then escort me out of the area.

The father's response to the gendarmerie ("the child is mine") represented his refusal to acknowledge the state-centered alignment between health officers and security forces as a legitimate force in regulating male circumcision on behalf of his son. In that instance, the state embodied by the gendarmerie failed to establish a contract with the father as the head of the family, sparking a moral conflict over the interests of the boy. Despite his lack of legal recognition, Sünnetçi Bülent could thus nevertheless successfully draw on long-standing communal acceptance and resist the threat of state violence.

The state-centered alignment's failure in gaining families' consent was unsurprisingly evident in Kurdish cities. Starting in the early twentieth century, the Turkish state sought to dominate Kurds without intermediaries such as tribal and religious solidarities, attempting to institute itself as the monopoly of the legitimate use of violence and shape mundane daily practices, such as the ways people talked and dressed, according to modern and national principles. An immediate consequence of the Turkification policies was the denial of Kurds' identity and political autonomy. As political scientist Senem Aslan (2015) writes:

> The state rulers perceived the strong authority of the local leaders such as religious sheikhs and tribal chiefs over the population to be an indication of backwardness as well as a serious constraint against establishing state authority. In the eyes of the state elite, these regions were associated with religious conservatism and reactionary politics, economic underdevelopment, socio-cultural backwardness, lawlessness, and an unruly population that was not familiar with state authority. (p. 38)

The oppression of Kurds and their resistance and uprisings against it continued after World War II. The 1960 coup legitimized and secured the role of the army in Turkish politics for decades to come by giving birth to the National Security Council, a government agency by which the military exercised a right of representation alongside the president of the Republic. Army generals as nonelected actors began to influence government policies and decisions about security issues—first and foremost, the Kurdish question. The Turkish military framed the question as a problem of "backwardness" in economic, social, and cultural senses rather than an ethnopolitical one (Yeğen 1999), thereby pressuring the government to launch the health care project in the Kurdish region as a way to assimilate the Kurds. The military interpreted the shortage of medical professionals in the region as a national security problem and envisioned the doctors' role as curing and caring for patients but also teaching Kurds basic principles of hygiene and "civilizing" them (Günal 2008). With this strategy, the military hoped to depoliticize Kurds.

However, the military's strategy of assimilation met with many problems, two of which are relevant to our discussion: first, health professionals, including health officers, were generally not eager to work in the region due to what they considered harsh living conditions (for instance, lack of basic infrastructure). Second, health professionals often reported the problem of not being able to communicate with locals in the region (Günal 2008). Policymakers briefly entertained the idea of providing a Kurdish language course for health professionals but never implemented it. This failure, far from being accidental, reflected how the Turkish state's ongoing and systematic colonizing Turkification policies sought to eradicate the public visibility and audibility of non-Turkish languages, particularly Kurdish (Aslan 2017).

For the above reasons, some of the health officers I interviewed mentioned that they had requested reassignment within five years of their first assignment in the Kurdish region. At the time of my research, itinerant circumcisers in the region outnumbered health officers and, contrary to what I observed in other regions, were largely concentrated at city centers rather than outskirts. These unlicensed itinerant circumcisers rarely had hostile interactions with health officers and were more comfortable talking to me about their experiences than the itinerant circumcisers in other regions. The Kurdish region's long history of opposition against the Turkish state's colonial and assimilationist policies enabled them to make extensive use of communal recognition and acceptance. The major impact on their practices came not so much from health officers as from the hospitals that have increasingly taken over the operations in recent decades in the Kurdish region and the other parts of the country.[9]

Itinerant circumcisers' reliance on local support within the Kurdish region and the rest of country does not, however, mean that they have continued performing circumcision in the same manner. On the contrary, the growing pressure of the medicalization of the 1960s had a profound impact on itinerant circumcisers, as it introduced new standards of care and transformed the normative understandings of circumciser (Sünnetçi) and circumcision.

PARTIAL IMITATIONS

Before medicalization, almost all itinerant circumcisers used straight razors to cut off the foreskin, and some applied herbs on the incision for postoperative care. Masters typically applied their own herbs and prepared them in advance with the help of their apprentices. Şamil described for me one of those medicines.

"My father was a very popular circumciser in the Southeast," Şamil said. Şamil's father learned to perform circumcision from his father, but Şamil himself never performed circumcision because he found it too stressful: "Some nights, my father could not sleep at all because he was too stressed out about the circumcisions he did a day before. After having seen that, I felt estranged from it." Şamil began to assist his father at a young age. During the summertime when school was not in session, he and his father traveled around the Kurdish region:

> There was no car, and we used to go from one village to another on the top of donkeys, camels, or horses. I used to get tips from locals, which I used as school pocket money. We were staying in the village overnight and then moving on to the next village early in the morning.

Şamil and his father used to circumcise at least fifty boys in each village. He carried his father's instrument bag, which contained a clamp for retracting the foreskin, a spindle for keeping it straight and stable, a straight razor for cutting it, and herbs for stopping the bleeding. The medicine consisted of a bitter herb (meyrankort)[10] and a small piece of bark that he and his father cut from a pine tree. The preparation involved crushing the bark into powder and then mixing it with the herb. Other itinerant circumcisers used ashes, animal dung, or medicine made from different kinds of herbs and tree barks. Two of my interviewees also mentioned that their fathers taught them how to make strings from animal intestines to stitch up the incisions.

As for pain management, some itinerant circumcisers put ice on children's groins before the operation, and a few of them applied a coolant spray, while others did not use anything. Some circumcisers also put a great deal of effort into cleaning their instruments for each circumcision. Şamil explained that he let his fathers' tools soak in a bowl of boiling water with the plastic parts of the tools outside the bowl. His father would then pick up the tools one by one, scrape the ragged edge of the scissors off by using the end of a pin, and then dry them off overnight at home before leaving for circumcision in the morning. Some itinerant circumcisers asked families to bring boiling water so that they could clean their instruments before the operations. Furthermore, a few of my interviewees used an open flame to sterilize their instruments at home in advance or cleaned their straight razors with alcohol after each operation. Others did not use any kind of sterilization method.

From the 1960s onwards, itinerant circumcisers were unevenly exposed to (professional) medicalization and its two main techniques: local anesthesia and sutures. In some parts of the country (for instance, northwestern Turkey), itinerant circumcisers initially spread rumors about what they considered to be "harmful" effects of local anesthesia and sutures on boys' health. These circumcisers warned families that the new techniques could cause impotence in their sons and that they should steer clear of health officers. By stitching the veins of a penis, some said, health officers were "stitching" their sons' masculinity. That said, all my interviewees were enthusiastic about adopting the new circumcision techniques—an opportunity that arose from their encounters with medical professionals.

Barber Ateş, who was born in 1936, began to perform circumcision in 1966. He learned it from his master, who was both a circumciser and a barber. Barber Ateş went to circumcisions with health officers and helped them find customers. In the meantime, he had also observed senior itinerant circumcisers, to whom he was grateful for improving his skills. However, he highlighted his encounters with medical professionals as a key turning point in the trajectory of his practice:

BARBER ATEŞ: We [he and his master] had been cutting it off without numbing it. Later, we started using Clordetyl [a coolant spray brand], the one used on football players. That helped us a little bit. We were cutting it off very quickly before the numbness wore off. My master was applying powder that he was making from . . . how should I say it? From the rotten parts of a tree, I think.

AUTHOR: Was he applying that after the operation?

BARBER ATEŞ: Yes, afterward. I used powder, too, but I got it from the pharmacy. I could not trust his powder. We continued using those methods for a long time. Then, I started using injections and sutures and applying sterilization.

AUTHOR: How did that happen?

BARBER ATEŞ: I had friends at a hospital here. The biggest favor they did for me was to teach me how to stitch up and dress a wound. Most of them are not alive anymore. May Allah be pleased with them [Allah rahmet eylesin]. I used to apply powder on penises after cutting off the foreskins and then wrap it with a bandage. That did not work well. It never stopped bleeding. Then, I learned how to do it properly. It was very simple: after cutting off the foreskin, you hold the vein with forceps, use absorbable catgut sutures, and then stitch it up. It heals very quickly. They also let me sterilize my instruments at their place.

AUTHOR: Were your friends health officers?

BARBER ATEŞ: Yes.

AUTHOR: When was this?

BARBER ATEŞ: Seventies. Seventy-five, I think. Local anesthesia made things much better, more comfortable. But some families at first were not happy with sutures because it was taking longer than it used to. I was aware of that. Sometimes they said "What kind of circumciser are you? It's been fifteen minutes and is still not over . . . the other master does it in a minute." I had a hearing problem. I still do, and I pretended that I did not hear them [he smiles].

Barber Ateş had always shown an abundance of concern toward the boys he circumcised. He watched other experienced circumcisers very carefully before starting to perform circumcision on his own. He used a coolant spray and powder to ease pain and suffering. His concerns about pain and harm facilitated his shift to (professional) medical techniques and skills that could, he thought, better deliver safe operations. As we shall see in the next chapter, however, not all families welcomed health officers' new circumcision techniques. And ironically, Ateş's adoption of modern circumcision blurred the distinction between himself and the health officers and sometimes sparked similarly negative reactions from families.

After my interview with Barber Ateş, I went to a nearby city on the same day by bus and met with Ferhat, who introduced me to another itinerant circumciser, Ceyhun, the next morning. Sünnetçi Ceyhun, born in 1930, had been performing circumcision for fifty years without a license. Like Barber Ateş, Sünnetçi Ceyhun had also learned to perform circumcision from his father and had similar encounters with medical professionals. Ferhat participated in our conversation as well:

CEYHUN: One day we went to a procedure, and I asked my father if I could do this on my own. He said "okay" and then watched me do it. This is how I started. I was traveling to six, seven villages by car within a day. My instruments included a clamp, a razor, and a spindle. I was pulling the foreskin like this [he uses my finger for illustration]. Sometimes, there was dirt on the foreskin and I was cleaning that first. Ours was practical [bizimki pratikti]; there was no injection at first. The injection came here later. Then, I started using it. I was using this herb called alışer. I used to dry it, mix it with the medicine I was getting from the pharmacy, and then apply it.

AUTHOR: Did you do that to stop the bleeding?

CEYHUN: Yes.

AUTHOR: And were you using a straight razor?

CEYHUN: Yes, I circumcised three generations here. Now, adult men sometimes come to me and want to kiss my hand.[11] I say, "I don't know you," then they say, "You circumcised me!"

AUTHOR: How did you learn to use local anesthesia?

CEYHUN: Doctors came here and showed me. They also showed me how to use sutures.

AUTHOR: Why did you want to learn the new methods?

CEYHUN: It was better for everyone. Kids don't cry, and I feel comfortable. But I also did not want to get into trouble.

AUTHOR: Trouble?

CEYHUN: Yes. Some families were asking if I was numbing it. But some families did not want me to use sutures. But what if it bled the next day? I did not have a license.

AUTHOR: Did you ever get into trouble?

CEYHUN: Not really. One day this health officer reported me, and then I told the prosecutor that this is a hoax, a health officers' hoax. Then, they let me go.

FERHAT: Sorry for interrupting. You know what? Health officers have a permit and can report others who do not have it. Because they want to make money and they see him as an obstacle.

AUTHOR: So, it happened more than once?

CEYHUN: Yes, but it is the same circumcision. Same skills, same methods.

Two major reasons motivated Sünnetçi Ceyhun to learn the surgical techniques: to better protect boys' well-being and to avoid state authorities. Yet, regardless of the reasons, a license, he believes, should not have been an issue at all. Health officers' hostile attitude toward him, in his and his friend's views, revealed nothing but the true economic motivation under the guise of altruistic interest in boys' well-being.[12] This is so because, as the reasoning goes, if health officers' true intentions were to protect boys' health, then they should have been contented with Sünnetçi Ceyhun's adoption of medical expertise. After all, Sünnetçi Ceyhun resentfully noted, "it is the same circumcision."

Mutually beneficial arrangements with health officers offered itinerant circumcisers an opportunity to incorporate the medical techniques as well. As the next chapter will show, health officers and itinerant circumcisers occasionally formed short-term cooperations whereby young and inexperienced health officers with no social networks observed itinerant circumcisers and benefitted from their social capital. The same arrangements also proved to be useful for itinerant circumcisers, for two reasons: first, when itinerant circumcisers performed circumcisions with health officers by their side and authorities inquired about permission, health officers could step forward, show their licenses, and act as a legal shield for itinerant circumcisers. When the roles were reversed, itinerant circumcisers could then have a chance to watch health officers and learn to use the surgical techniques.

Furthermore, some itinerant circumcisers were self-taught in using medical techniques. With no clue as to where to apply the injection at first, these circumcisers learned and improved their skills by trial and error. Many of them reported that they began wanting to incorporate local anesthesia because families who had seen it used in circumcisions started asking for it. Some also praised the new method for easing pain more effectively. As one of them said: "You should always be open to novelties."

Other itinerant circumcisers learned the surgical techniques and skills from their superiors during compulsory military services (though, as we shall see in the next chapter, this option was more widely available to health officers). Sünnetçi Coşku, a fifty-one-year-old barber, completed his seventeen-month-long military service in Ankara, where he also learned to perform medicalized techniques. He and I talked at his barbershop as he was cutting his customer's hair. I asked him about his training:

AUTHOR: When did you start working as a barber?

COŞKU: We were a big family. We were ten siblings, plus my parents, so twelve people. We were poor. I did not finish school. I finished middle school, though. I started as an apprentice when I was six years old. I extracted teeth in the past, too. My master was also performing circumcision.

AUTHOR: Did you watch him?

COŞKU: Yes, I did. But his method was different from mine. His method was old. There was no numbing or stitching. But at first, I traveled around with my master.

AUTHOR: What is your method?

COŞKU: Mine is fenni. I learned it in the military. I was at a hospital with eighty beds. They [doctors] were circumcising uncircumcised soldiers, and I was assisting them. I was cleaning and dressing the incision. I now circumcise with sutures and anesthesia.

AUTHOR: How did families react to these methods?

COŞKU: Some of them complained, because it was taking too long. With sutures, it can take ten minutes longer. With the old method, you cut it off and then wrapped it up. That's it. It is, of course, ridiculous that they were complaining. Why would you get your hand burned when you have tongs, right?

AUTHOR: Do you remember your first circumcision?

COŞKU: I do. It was simple. Oh, and I always ask families before circumcision if their boys have any illness like hepatitis or something.

AUTHOR: What happens if they have?

COŞKU: I send them to a hospital.

Military service in Turkey served as a site where uncircumcised soldiers were sometimes circumcised—a routine that enabled a few itinerant circumcisers like Sünnetçi Coşku to acquire (professional) medical expertise and promote medical values, goals, and principles in male circumcision. Sünnetçi Coşku was assigned to a military hospital, where he learned the medical techniques and gained literacy in medicine, as shown by his emphasis on both the scientific nature of his techniques and his knowledge about medical illnesses that can complicate the operations.

Overall, we can identify three main reasons behind itinerant circumcisers' desires to learn the surgical techniques: (a) families' growing demands for these techniques, (b) potential problems with state authorities, and (c) moral concerns about boys' well-being. In light of the health officers' challenges faced by itinerant circumcisers starting in the 1960s, performing circumcision increasingly signified a risk of violating the 1928 law and of transgressing the medicalized notion of a safe procedure—a notion that itinerant circumcisers embraced, too. Accordingly, to circumvent the state-backed medical authority, a varying degree of communal support and traditional authority enabled unlicensed itinerant circumcisers to sustain their practices and maintain their distinction from their rivals while also imitating them thanks to mostly informal and sporadic encounters with medical professionals.

Nonetheless, unlike in other contexts such as India (Langford 2012) and China (Lei 2014) where non-Western modalities of healing and medicine enjoyed an organizational basis (for instance, schools), itinerant circumcisers were in no position to collectively challenge the Turkish medico-bureaucratic authority. Except for two itinerant circumcisers, none of my interviewees had trained their sons for circumcision, and those trained by their fathers represented the last generation of itinerant circumcisers. Health officers, thus, have gradually replaced itinerant circumcisers, albeit in a geographically uneven manner.

MEDICALIZATION BEYOND PROFESSIONALISM

The modern and national discourse behind the state-led medicalization of male circumcision dismissed itinerant circumcisers for their supposed lack of concern for boys' well-being. This discourse has also informed much of the academic writing on medicine that focuses on these practitioners. Analyzing forty cases of circumcision complications (for instance, severe bleeding, infections, and inadequate removal of foreskin) in Turkey, Latifoglu et al. (1999) argue that in all but three cases, boys were circumcised by "a medically unqualified traditional itinerant circumciser" (p. 87). Similarly, the urologist

Özdemir (1997) reports that, over a ten year period (1987–1997), 220 cases with complications visited the emergency room or outpatient departments at a hospital located in the Kurdish region. He shows that 85 percent of the patients with complications were circumcised by traditional circumcisers. These studies hold itinerant circumcisers responsible for boys' suffering.

Unfortunately, such studies disseminate the dominant stereotype of the itinerant circumciser without asking the critical question of why some families continued having their sons circumcised by itinerant circumcisers. Meanwhile, many health officers I interviewed provided an overly simple and biased answer to this question: families' ignorance (cehalet). Yet, as this chapter has shown, it is trust, rather than ignorance as a so-called cultural trait, that has been the crucial factor in some families' sustained preference for itinerant circumcisers. These families did not acknowledge the state and its incarnations, such as health officers and security forces, as legitimate and instead continued to work with the group of circumcisers with whom they forged ties over generations. Moreover, this chapter has proved that families were knowledgeable about the benefits of new medical techniques, as some pressured itinerant circumcisers to incorporate them. Their problem was not with the medical techniques per se but those who used them.

Contrary to studies that posit an overly neat distinction between itinerant circumcisers and health professionals, our discussion in this chapter has shown that itinerant circumcisers, though largely excluded from the medico-bureaucratic apparatus, imitated health officers and learned, to some degree, medical circumcision techniques, knowledge, and skills while also upholding their own traditional authority. Itinerant circumcisers' ambivalent attachment to the medicalization process served as a safeguard against the total annihilation of the boundary between themselves and health officers who stigmatized them. Itinerant circumcisers simultaneously incorporated what they disavowed, which often generated both resentment and anger toward health officers and admiration for their techniques.

In an analysis of the medicalization of childbirth on a Guatemalan plantation, the anthropologist Sheila Cosminsky (2016) describes how midwives and doctors use both a local ethno-obstetric model and a biomedical model of birth to establish authoritative knowledge about birth and pregnancy. While the former regards pregnancy and birth as "resulting in an imbalance of hot and cold qualities and representing a normal but potentially dangerous state" (p. 2), the latter views them as a physiological disturbance and an abnormal state. Yet, in the case of male circumcision in Turkey, no ethnomedical model preceded the biomedical model, and itinerant circumcisers were therefore eager to embrace the latter in a contradictory manner.

As the sociologist Gil Eyal (2013) argues, professionals seeking to establish a monopoly over their expertise may obstruct the expansion of medicalization within society by excluding potential interlopers from their field who could otherwise participate in the medicalization process. The medicalization of male circumcision in Turkey offered a case where such interlopers, to some extent, countered medical professionals' monopoly, not to reject but rather to embrace their medical expertise. Furthermore, some doctors and health officers, rather than excluding itinerant circumcisers, taught them the surgical techniques because they thought that their support would eventually be beneficial to the boys the itinerant circumcisers would circumcise. In doing so, these doctors and health officers attached themselves to their medical expertise in a way that fostered collaboration across practitioners. The findings of the chapter thus suggest that boys in Turkey would greatly benefit from the systematic incorporation of itinerant circumcisers into the medico-bureaucratic network, as they would expand the range of biomedical care.

As I conversed with Sünnetçi Orhan at his clinic in a medium-sized city in central Anatolia, he got a phone call from a family who wanted to have their son circumcised that day. Sünnetçi Orhan agreed, adding that he had a guest at his clinic who might come with him. He hung up and said the family would let him bring me along. He quickly packed his circumcision instruments, and within a few minutes, I was in the car of a man I'd met less than an hour earlier, driving to a family home where he would perform circumcision. Our conversation continued during our short ride.

Sünnetçi Orhan was a fifty-six-year-old health officer and had been performing circumcision for thirty-two years. He was one of the few Turkish health officers I met who also traveled to other countries (including Sudan, Somalia, Kenya, and Georgia) for circumcisions sponsored by Muslim civil society organizations. He told me that he had wanted to get into this business for social as well as financial reasons, as he enjoyed the intimate interactions with people: "I have been doing this for years, and there is no household that I've not been in. So, this was a good fit for me." As we were driving from the city center to the outskirts, I asked him about his encounters with families and itinerant circumcisers when he first started performing circumcision in 1972:

ORHAN: Every region used to have its own circumcisers. There were Abdals [a group of itinerant circumcisers] in this city. These circumcisers learned it from their fathers and were using old methods. Of course, our method was different and is still being used. We were numbing it. No pain, no blood—this method was embraced by people. Thus, old circumcisers disappeared. They all died.

AUTHOR: Was there any tension between you and the Abdals?

ORHAN: No, not really. I did not interact with them [onlarla muhatap olmadim].

We were buzzed into the building, where the family lived on the first floor, and greeted by a mother, a father, their seven-year-old son dressed in a circumcision outfit, and a grandfather who guided us to the living room. Sünnetçi Orhan placed his white portable stretcher on the floor and had the boy—who looked rather subdued—lie down on it. He then opened a kit containing the health officer's standard tools: needles, sutures, scissors, scalpel, and forceps (some health officers I observed used thermal cautery, instead of a scalpel, to cut off the foreskin). As he prepared a local anesthetic, he told me that although he had worked with assistants in the past, he was now working alone, and he liked it. "I don't like managing people," he added.

He then injected an anesthetic into the boy's groin area, and while waiting for it to take effect, he started chatting with the boy's eighty-four-year-old grandfather. We learned that the grandfather had been an itinerant circumciser; he had performed circumcision for decades but retired several years previously. Sünnetçi Orhan asked the grandfather if he would instead want to circumcise his grandson (during my research many practitioners told me proudly that they had circumcised their sons and grandsons, seeing it as a form of intergenerational intimacy). The grandfather shook his head to indicate no; his hands were too shaky for safe circumcision. Sünnetçi Orhan asked him about his experience of performing male circumcision:

ORHAN: How did you circumcise kids in the past?
GRANDFATHER: I learned to use local anesthesia at some point.
ORHAN: Oh, really?
GRANDFATHER: Yeah, and we used to use sutures made from animal intestines. A
    doctor taught me how to apply local anesthesia.

The boy's groin was now sufficiently numbed. Scalpel in hand, Sünnetçi Orhan turned to the family members, asking them to hold the boy tight so that he could start the operation. Restraining boys during the procedure is a mode of care for both boys and circumcisers, as both are otherwise at risk of harm: sudden moves can make scalpels slip, damaging penises or circumcisers' hands. All three family members looked at each other, each hoping to delegate the task to someone else. I would witness similar hesitation in many other faces over the course of my research: family members seemed disturbed at being asked to take an active part in what is often perceived as a potentially painful operation. Agreeing to share in restraining a boy could also mean assuming responsibility for the pain he might feel during circumcision. Yet, they also knew that refusing could result in injury to their (grand)sons. Hence, their ambivalence toward the call.

The mother finally volunteered, but Sünnetçi Orhan said that one person was insufficient. With no other relative stepping forward, Sünnetçi Orhan turned to me for help. The mother and I held down the boy—who now looked scared—as Sünnetçi Orhan began to cut some of the foreskin off, reassuring the boy that he would not feel pain. The mother and father turned their heads away and closed their eyes while Sünnetçi Orhan described the operation to me as he proceeded. Meanwhile, the grandfather tried to distract the boy by talking to him and making him laugh. After cutting off the foreskin, Sünnetçi Orhan quickly moved to feeling the incision with his fingers to find bleeding spots and stitching them using absorbable sutures. After a few shrieks from the boy, Sünnetçi Orhan completed the procedure and instructed the mother regarding postoperative care: no showering for twenty-four hours and pain-killers could be used if necessary.

When juxtaposed with his remarks about Abdals from our car ride, Sünnetçi Orhan's surprise about the grandfather using local anesthesia reveals a deeper dilemma unique to the medicalization of male circumcision during the 1960s. His remarks repeated the dominant male circumcision narrative that presumed a clear-cut distinction between health officers as agents of medicalization and itinerant circumcisers. Yet, as the previous chapter showed, itinerant circumcisers like the grandfather had adopted what health officers regarded as an essential component of the medicalized circumcision and thus blurred the distinction between themselves and health officers.

This chapter analyzes the medicalization of male circumcision during the developmentalist era from the perspective of health officers. With the establishment of the Turkish Republic in the early twentieth century, especially as the state-led developmentalist era began in the 1960s, painless circumcision became a biopolitical goal of protecting boys' health. It emerged as a tool for professional control and status, and a new locus of moral optimism for the future that was embedded within the secular, national, and modern imagination. As state-authorized practitioners, health officers like Orhan became dual agents in this era: they acted simultaneously as moral pioneers of medicalized circumcision and as state agents who expanded state power over a new social field. They framed circumcision pain as acute and localizable within the body and held that it was caused by organic and physiological dysfunctions. And to manage this pain, they introduced the two techniques of local anesthesia and sutures,[1] plus medical hygiene, regular follow-ups, professional skills, and medical knowledge and discourse.

Health officers strove to medicalize the practice and gain families' trust in new surgical techniques. However, performing circumcision was associated with itinerant circumcisers known as Sünnetçi, who were, as we saw in chapter 1, stigmatized in health officers' eyes (and medical professionals' eyes in general) but were well respected in communities. How then could health officers differentiate themselves from itinerant circumcisers, represent themselves as moral pioneers, and render performing circumcision a site of professional prestige, all while garnering trust from families accustomed to sünnetçi? How could they avoid being mistaken for sünnetçi as well as failing to secure a footing in communities—both of which would lead to the dissolution of their identity as practitioners? How did they confront the pressure associated with the stigmatized position of sünnetçi?

The chapter argues that health officers sustained an ambivalent relationship with Sünnetçi as they transformed themselves into Fenni Sünnetçi (the Scientific Circumciser). Fenni Sünnetçi invoked science and medicine while remaining relevant to families. The term refers to a compromised and contradictory subject formation wherein health officers incorporated what they otherwise disavowed: Sünnetçi. In doing so, they shielded themselves against the risk of a complete breakdown of the boundary between traditional practitioners and themselves, while also partially identifying with Sünnetçi. Fenni Sünnetçi, in other words, represented a new professional subjectivity emerging from the reorganization of male circumcision under a medical authority, based on the dispossession and exclusion of rural communities' practitioners. It assumed a proper balance in relation to itinerant circumcisers—a balance that animated and coordinated health officers' desire for medicalization.

In what follows, I first situate the medicalization of male circumcision within a broader transformation of society and polity that began after the establishment of the Turkish Republic in 1923. Bringing male circumcision under state control was consistent with the new Turkish ruling elites' aspirations for modernizing the society and constructing a Turkish "culture" that was different from what they imagined as "Western." However, the medico-bureaucratic expansion did not occur in everyday life until the 1960s, when the Turkish state launched a program that recruited health officers as part of the medical team responsible for delivering health care services, including medical male circumcision.

The following sections examine health officers' status-related concerns as they sought to medicalize the practice and show how they managed these concerns through binding themselves to fenni sünnetçi: a self-transformation from health officers, a group of inexperienced yet state-authorized and medically-trained practitioners with no preexisting ties to communities, into fenni sünnetçi, experienced practitioners recognized by the communities they served. Paradoxically, the emergence of fenni sünnetçi as drivers of medicalization rested on both the avowal and disavowal of their similarity to the itinerant circumcisers who had been serving families for generations.

The medicalization of male circumcision in the post–World War II period relied upon the broadening capacity of a medico-bureaucratic apparatus that employed health officers and other medical professionals. However, while the 1928 law rendered health officers eligible for performing circumcisions, no regulatory supervision over health officers' activities existed, even in the 1960s. Health officers had full discretionary power over whether to begin to perform circumcisions, and the reality that almost every Muslim boy in Turkey gets circumcised made circumcision-for-fee an enticing option for state-authorized health officers. Yet, without the transformation of health officers into fenni sünnetçi, as I argue below, neither the alluring economic opportunity nor the massive network of health care established during the developmentalist era could have brought the practice under the state-medical authority.

THE 1920S–1950S

Although Ottoman surgeons introduced medical techniques to male circumcision in the late nineteenth century, the impact of medicine on male circumcision during that era, as shown in chapter 3, remained confined to imperial circumcisions. Only with the establishment of the Turkish Republic did the medicalization of male circumcision begin to influence the wider population.

Starting in 1923, the Turkish ruling elites (military officers, politicians, bureaucrats, and internationally trained doctors) sought to reorganize social, political, and economic structures inherited from the Empire. The late Ottoman Empire in the nineteenth century and the young Turkish Republic in the early twentieth were both beset by aggressive external European polities that incorporated modern techniques of discipline and governmentality (such as military engineering, medicine, sanitation, and hygiene). In the eyes of the Turkish elites, the Ottoman Empire, having lasted more than six centuries, owed its eventual dismantling to its failure to keep pace in adopting these techniques—a failure that facilitated the establishment of European dominance in the Muslim world. Reforms proposed in the late empire and early republican periods thus entailed "the production and application of new kinds of knowledge which existing institutions were not producing but which has to be gleaned from elsewhere" (Silverstein 2003, p. 508). Authority and prestige were relocated from Islamic and traditional knowledges to scientific knowledge and authorities.[2] Turkish elites aimed to cultivate new identities based on (a) new institutions such as the conjugal family and the military, (b) new loyalties (to the national and secular state), and (c) a new philosophical ground (particularly science and positivism).

Although neither the Ottoman Empire nor Turkey was ever colonized—and should, on the contrary, be seen as colonizing forces themselves—elites' perspective on postindependence Turkey was fraught with uncertainties like those observed in postcolonial contexts. How could the Turkish nation imitate the (imagined) West and be part of the Western or modern world without compromising its distinct (imagined) identity? Ziya Gökalp, the main ideologue of the official Turkish nationalism (Kemalism) in the early twentieth century, proposed a distinction between civilization (technology, science, and knowledge) and culture (a set of values and habits), warning against the risk of over-Westernization. "Too much" Westernization, he argued, would lead to moral corruption and cultural decay. He instead suggested that Turkey should embrace the material aspects of the civilization of the West while protecting and developing "authentic" and "pure" Turkish national culture (Kadioğlu 1996).

Accordingly, in the ensuing years of the establishment of the Republic, the ruling elites reevaluated the practices, beliefs, and forms of knowledge characteristic of the Ottoman past and modified (or eliminated, if necessary) those based on perceived compatibility—or incompatibility—with the Westernized civilization and the Turkish cultural identity. The new governmental, military, and intellectual leaders denigrated and banned practices like religious healing (Dole 2004, 2012) and fortune-telling (Korkman 2015b), as these practices, the leaders claimed, held the Ottoman Empire back and obstructed Turkey's national progress and development in a global modern world. In the field of health and health care, modern techniques, discourses, and knowledge were initially confined to the army but gradually and unevenly expanded to the wider society. As Turkey's political climate changed, medical professionals became the face of the modern state, charging its political power with the civilizational ethos of biomedical authority, knowledge, and techniques.

Adding to the ideological and administrative challenges faced by elites was Turkey's increasingly urgent population crisis in the aftermath of a series of wars (the Balkan Wars in 1912–1913, World War I, and the Independence War) and epidemics, including tuberculosis, syphilis, and typhus (Shorter 1985). Half of Turkey's twelve million people were malaria-stricken, and around a million people suffered from tuberculosis (Günal 2008). The wars occasioned a significant loss of the male population, exacerbated by an alarming increase in infant and child mortality rates.[3] Associating demographic strength with economic and military power, the Turkish state aimed at improving the health of the new nation's citizens. Until the end of World War II, the regime thus pursued pronatalist policies and sanitary reform, toward the paired goals of increasing the size of the nation's population and improving the health of its citizens. The Penal Code of 1926 that made abortion illegal and the Law of Public Health of 1930 were both meant to enable the government to increase the birth rate and prevent deaths from diseases (Günal 2008).

The state also prohibited importing, producing, or selling contraceptives and supported families with children. The Ministry of Health and Social Assistance allocated funds to identify mothers with more than six children and provide grants to them. By 1960, Turkey's total population was close to twenty-eight million (Yilmaz 2015). Furthermore, scientifically trained doctors began to act as the agents of modernization, responsible for improving the health of Anatolia's population and teaching people how to live according to modern scientific norms (such as Western hygiene). New laws addressed the problems of epidemics and child mortality and decreed that health workers should be trained in public health. For the nationalist ideology, medicine and health became, therefore, essential to crafting modern and healthy subjects.

The state's involvement in male circumcision in the initial decades of the Republic should be considered in the context of this rise of the nationalist, modern, and secular vision of the society as well as practical concerns about a war-torn and epidemic-ridden population. Indeed, children's well-being and health were important considerations in the new biopolitical rationality, for it concerned itself with the future of the population. Modern and nationalist elites designated themselves as the guardians of Turkey's children and regarded the health of those children as too important to be left in the hands of "incompetent" practitioners. Itinerant circumcisers faced stigmatization for using techniques deemed detrimental to children's well-being. As a contributor to the journal *Ülkü* wrote:[4]

> Altogether ignorant and foul would-be midwives are birthing our mother's children and of course, killing most of them . . . Under the name of surgery, inexperienced operators are treating people with wounds, sprains, and broken bones, and they are leaving most handicapped . . . The calamities that ignorant midwives, would-be surgeons, dentist barbers, and circumcisers found in the coffee-house-corner offices have been producing for years have passed before us. (1933, p. 255)

Accordingly, rather than banning male circumcision as they had banned religious healing and fortune-telling, the Turkish state in 1928 brought the medical aspects of the practice under its purview. The Republican People's Party (CHP) issued the Law on the Application of Medicine and its Branches (Tababet ve Şuabatı San'atlarının Tarzı İcrasına Dair Kanun).[5] The law proclaimed that practicing medicine, including male circumcision, would be limited only to those who graduated from the Turkish faculties of medicine or those with equivalent degrees approved by the Ministry of Health and Social Aid. In doing so, the state codified male circumcision as a medical procedure to be performed only by practitioners with medical degrees and licenses. The law carried penalties of up to a month of prison time or small fines for unlicensed practitioners who did not comply with the restrictions and, as a result, posed a risk to children's health.

That said, the law did not preclude controversies over male circumcision among doctors with sharply polarized perspectives about male circumcision. Pediatrician Kadri Raşit Anday was among the doctors who opposed male circumcision whether medicalized or not. After three years of studying medicine at the Imperial Military School of Medicine (Mekteb-i Tıbbiye-i Şahane) in Istanbul, Anday dropped out of school and went to Paris to complete his studies under the supervision of the French physiologist Charles Richet. He returned to Istanbul in 1901 and became a professor at the Imperial Civil Medical School (Mekteb-i Tıbbiye-yi Mülkiye). During the first years of the Republic, he was involved in the debate over male circumcision as a passionate opponent:

> Inflammation is not a good reason for circumcision. There was no water in Arabia and our prophet was born circumcised. Europeans shower every day. Turks are now part of the Western civilization and when you shower, you don't need circumcision. (Ataseven 2005, 43)

Another doctor, the psychiatrist Nazım Şakir, agreed with Anday that the practice should be banned:

> Circumcision is not medically necessary. Considering that there is no circumcision in civilized nations, it is inappropriate for us to take a step backward and perform circumcision. Both circumcised and uncircumcised men can be filthy. There are many uncircumcised Europeans who are clean. The foreskin is a gift from nature and circumcision means cutting this gift off. (Ataseven 2005, 44)

These health professionals believed that if the state was seeking to catch up with the European level of civilization, then male circumcision should not be practiced at all except for in circumstances where it was medically necessary. Criticizing the association between health and male circumcision, they argued that basic hygienic routines (for instance, daily showers) could protect boys from the diseases that male circumcision was claimed to prevent.

Other doctors, however, offered counterarguments highlighting the health benefits of male circumcision. The orthopedist Orhan Abdi, who had studied medicine in Germany in 1900, argued that circumcision would prevent syphilis (Ataseven 2005; Topuzlu 1935). The pro-circumcision doctors proposed that, rather than prohibiting the practice, the state should exercise strict surveillance over practitioners and eliminate those without licenses. Some also emphasized

the religious significance of male circumcision for Muslims, who now constituted the majority of the population in the post–Ottoman Empire era. For
pro-circumcision doctors, the modernized (that is, medicalized) form of male
circumcision was not only compatible with the ethos of civilization but also
crucial for constructing a national identity infused with, but not mastered by,
(Sunni) Islam.

The debate among health professionals took a critical turn when Cemil
Topuzlu, an internationally recognized surgeon, brought the issue to the Turkish Medical Research Council (Türkiye Tıp Encümeni) in 1934 and delivered
a presentation titled "Is circumcision beneficial to health?" (Sünnet Sağlık
İçin Faydalı mıdır?). Topuzlu had studied medicine in Paris and had served
in 1919 as a minister of development during the late Ottoman Empire. In his
presentation, he took issue with pro-circumcision arguments, noting that the
Quran does not mention male circumcision. He said:

> Let us focus on the hygienic aspect of circumcision. It is argued that a cir-
> cumcised man does not need to worry about hygiene. Is this not a strange
> argument for avoiding personal hygiene? Don't people normally wash every
> part of their bodies one by one? Why should they not bother doing the same
> thing for their reproductive organs [tenasül aletleri]? Are we lower than
> animals in this respect? There is no reason to cut off an important part of
> the reproductive organ to avoid performing daily self-care that takes only
> a couple of seconds. Should we also cut off our toes so that we would not
> need to trim or clean our toenails? (Topuzlu 1935, p. 6)

Although Topuzlu did not go so far as to advocate outlawing circumcision, he
recommended that the council prepare a bill prohibiting circumcision before
age eighteen and send it to the Ministry of Health and Social Aid. At the
same time, the debate among doctors over male circumcision expanded beyond the medical community and made headlines. Laypeople expressed their
views in opinion pieces in newspapers, largely criticizing the anti-circumcision
camp for its vulgar imitation of the West and for moving away from Islamic
traditions.

For the medical community and public alike, the debate over male circumcision would become yet another site where the broader concern about
the boundaries between "civilization" and "culture," the constitutive dichotomy
of the official Turkish modern identity, played itself out. More specifically, if
"foreskins are facts—cultural facts whether removed or retained" (Boon 1995,
p. 556), then in the early years of the Republic young boys' foreskins in Turkey
symbolically became part of major issues such as modernization, secularism,
and nationalism. Ideologically, a modernized male circumcision signified a

proper distance from, and yet safe proximity to, the imagined "West": continuing the practice would serve as a safeguard against "over-Westernization," while the pragmatic appropriation of modern techniques would support Turkey's claim to belong to the modern world.

Topuzlu's bill was never prepared, the circumcision clause of the 1928 law remained in place until 2015 (see chapter 5), and the debate over the necessity of circumcision soon gave way to the problematization of circumcision methods and instruments, as doctors and public health authorities responded to reports of circumcision injuries and accidents. Health professionals laid these cases at the feet of itinerant circumcisers who, as we saw in chapter 1, had no place in the Turkish nation's self-representation.

THE 1960s–1980s

Circumcision is no longer a nightmare for children. Children cheerfully run around after being circumcised in the blink of an eye. Elderly men who recall the sweet yet frightening memories of their circumcisions watch these circumcisions in awe and feel sorry and regret they were born too early. Owing to the new medical techniques [local anesthesia and sutures] children only noticed the completion of their circumcision hours after the operation. It is now impossible to see a child crying in front of circumcisers, and children who can put their pants back on right after the operation can mingle with their friends and act like nothing happened. Circumcisions from ten, twenty years ago are now history. (*Hürriyet*, July 1, 1977)

Here a health officer, quoted in a widely-read mainstream Turkish newspaper in 1977, captures health officers' efforts to portray the medical circumcision techniques to the public as morally desirable, charged with an "aura of benevolence" (Taussig 1980, 4). Joyfully proclaiming the inauguration of a new era ("Circumcisions from ten, twenty years ago are now history"), however exaggerated that might sound, the speaker recasts itinerant circumcisers' techniques as relics of the past that caused unnecessary pain and suffering in boys. In reshaping the public discourse on circumcision, health officers presented themselves as the main actors promising families painless and safe circumcisions. For instance, health officers claimed to leave behind the widespread custom of covering the newly circumcised penises with a circumcision hat for hours, or of keeping pants off for days until the incision was healed. With the help of the medical techniques, boys, they highlighted, could now "put their pants back on" right away after the operation, without worrying that their clothing would rub against the healing incision.

The health officers' self-confidence was, in part, based on their key role in the expansion of state-delivered health care in the 1960s. Following the 1960 coup d'état, the 1961 Turkish Constitution affirmed health care as a fundamental citizenship right and charged the medico-bureaucratic apparatus with the provision of preventive and curative care for citizens. After the military ceded power later the same year, the goal of improving the health of the population made its way into the agenda of civilian governments. Although the financial structure for health care services never ceased to be a matter of dispute, the governments of the 1960s (and beyond) agreed that establishing a public health care infrastructure was the right organizational model for optimal health care delivery. This model, it was thought, could solve the rural-urban gap in access to health care services and public health measures.

The health care infrastructure was composed of health posts and stations located in cities, towns, and villages. Health stations each served a population of 2500–3000 and consisted of a midwife who took care of maternal and child health. Each health post served a population of 5,000–10,000 in rural areas and 14,000–35,000 in urban areas. These posts employed a general practitioner, a nurse, a midwife, a health officer, a medical secretary, a driver, and a janitor. The organizational goals were the integration of health care services, the restructuring of the referral chain, the strengthening of primary care services (which would eventually reduce the burden on hospitals), and the transformation of citizens' habitual comportment concerning medicine, health, and healing. According to the plan, a citizen's first contact with the medical system would not be the hospital but a health clinic, where the patient could be diagnosed and receive life-saving medicines free of charge (Günal 2008). The medical staff (general practitioners, nurses, midwives, and health officers) were to monitor the population and carry out tasks such as home visits to provide both preventive and curative services, including keeping medical records, administering vaccination, prescribing drugs, and providing prenatal care and first aid. These medical teams would also teach citizens modern health principles, including hygiene, and elicit their cooperation in improving their health (Aksakoğlu 2008).

The health care project of the 1960s extended the preexisting health care infrastructure significantly, albeit not evenly.[6] Health officers, along with other medical actors, were assigned as primary care providers.[7] These low-ranked male professionals (underneath doctors and equivalent in status to nurses, who were exclusively female) joined the health care workforce in their late teens or early twenties after completing high school and became subordinate members of the centralized Turkish public administration. Equipped with scientific credentials and institutional prestige, they began to perform various medical tasks, including administering vaccinations, providing first aid, and performing circumcision, though not all health officers performed circumcision for the reasons discussed below. Health officers held a secure bureaucratic position that came with stable income and generous pension benefits. Like other civil servants in Turkey, health officers were banned from engaging in for-profit commercial or trade activities, to ensure the use of their energies, skills, and time for the public good (Kapucu and Palabıyık 2008). However, it was (and still is) very common in Turkey for low-level civil servants to engage in jobs on the side for untaxed additional income. Local state authorities either turn a blind eye to these activities or lack the logistical capacity to monitor them. From the gray area at the intersection of circumcision's legal status and the duties and responsibilities of the health officer emerged an opportunity for health officers to earn fees by performing circumcision.

FENNI SÜNNETÇI

People were ignorant. A man who was bitten by a snake would go to a local healer rather than a doctor. They did not believe in doctors. A snake once bit a man's wife, and I prevented him from taking her to a local healer. I told him to take his wife to a hospital; otherwise, I would report him to the police.

Thus eighty-five-year-old Hüsnü, a retired health officer assigned to a town in western Turkey in 1958, described his early encounters with locals. The observations he shared with me over a long conversation were fraught with a duality concerning köylü [peasants]. He complained that the locals did not initially use his circumcision services and preferred traditional circumcisers over him. Yet he also emphasized that families were smart enough to eventually realize the benefits of the medical techniques. He described rural people as sly, ignorant, brutish, and narrow-minded, but also as caring and hardworking, and this duality appeared in many of my conversations with other health officers as well.

The success of health officers' endeavor to medicalize male circumcision hinged on gaining legitimacy and recognition from the public for their new ways of understanding, reflecting on, and probing into the nonmedical phenomenon of circumcision. This question of recognition becomes an especially thorny one when medicalization is of a top-down and noncooperative nature. One can, of course, claim that medicalization is never simply a seamless, unidirectional, and homogenous process, since it often unfolds unevenly and generates a variety of responses, including cooperation, accommodation, and contestation.[8] However, such conflicts have tended to be augmented by state-led medicalization and modernization based on the strategy of usurpation and the rigid binaries of nationalist ideology such as modern versus traditional, knowledge versus ignorance, or science versus religion. This ideology simultaneously posits the population as an object of social engineering and a potential obstacle to national progress and development. At the same time, the same "ignorant" individual members of the population control the fate of medicalization, for they are the ones who would confer recognition on the medical claims. And this inevitable dependence on local recognition renders health officers' attitude toward performing male circumcision ambivalent—an attitude often colored with a sense of bitterness.

The central government assigned health officers to different parts of the country, and many health officers requested reassignment to a different location after a few years (as mentioned in the previous chapter). Some of them started performing circumcisions at their first locations, but others did not. As indicated above, a civil servant position in Turkey in the post–World War II period came with job security, relatively generous access to health care, and a decent pension. Yet, depending on the region's level of economic development and the number of active circumcisers in the area, performing circumcision could still be quite a lucrative option for them. By performing circumcision as a source of extra income, some health officers were able to achieve a standard of living that would otherwise have been out of their reach. Some of my informants mentioned that the income they earned from circumcision helped them send their children to college and even to study abroad. Others pointed out to me the properties (buildings, houses, or land) they had bought with the proceeds of their circumcision practices.

Despite the potential personal financial benefits, not all health officers wanted to perform circumcision, because they did not want to be mistaken for sünnetçi. Others who did end up going into the business recalled being initially uncomfortable with the decision. Tevfik, a fifty-five-year-old health officer, at first did not want to perform circumcision because, he said, "Abdals, you know, gypsies [*çingeneler*] were doing it.[9] I did not want to be called 'sünnetçi.'" When I asked him whether he ever traveled around for circumcision, he got upset: "No! I am not a gypsy. I worked only by appointment."

Ali, another health officer around the same age as Tevfik, was also initially reluctant to start performing circumcision. Sünnetçi Ali finished his medical training in 1961 and began to perform circumcision only in 1980. When I asked him about the time gap, he said:

> I have been doing this since 1980. Before that, we [health officers] were not inclined to do it because of Abdals. It was seen as a job for Abdals. Then, we, as health officers, said, "We should take it over." We thought ours was better

and healthier, and to be honest, it paid well. So we did it because people wanted circumcision to be medical and it also made sense economically.

Neither the potential economic returns nor the publicized benefits of modern circumcision sufficed to motivate Ali to start his own practice. He had been working at a health post and delivering medical services for the community. Among these services, circumcision occupied an ambiguous position in his habitus: it was not a typical medical service, as it was performed by traditional circumcisers whom he disdained. For him, Sünnetçi was saturated with conflicting meanings, values, and emotions.

Regardless of where and when they began to perform circumcision, health officers without preexisting ties to locals encountered the tension between their goal to achieve widespread popular acceptance and their need to maintain the professional prestige that set them apart from nonprofessionals. Whereas in the context of their medical training male circumcision had been a medical operation that carried professional prestige, in the towns and rural communities wherein health officers settled, male circumcision was strongly associated with itinerant circumcisers who had been serving communities for generations. Health officers' desire for recognition, acceptance, and trust from the public led them to an impasse and, consequently, to complex identificatory processes. First, health officers who wished to gain public acceptance had to identify the lowest common denominator that would render them immediately legible and legitimate in the eyes of the public. This denominator was identifying as sünnetçi. Yet, the choice to identify as sünnetçi involved risk: the risk of collapsing the boundaries between themselves and the itinerant circumcisers, which would threaten to damage the health officers' professional (self-)image. It was the same risk that alienated those health officers who never began to perform circumcision.

Starting in the 1960s, health officers popularized the terms "fenni sünnet" (scientific circumcision) and "fenni sünnetçi" (scientific circumciser), both of which date to the late Ottoman period (Yılmaz 2019). These labels showed up not only in newspapers but also on the streets of cities and towns, where health officers began to hand out or post on walls flyers that promoted their services. Some health officers later opened clinics advertised under the name "fenni sünnetçi," where they provided male circumcision services alongside other services such as measuring blood pressure, providing first aid, administering injections, and even piercing ears. However, most health officers performed circumcision at families' homes.

Fenni sünnetçi emerged as a response to the dilemma health officers faced in their attempts to medicalize male circumcision. On the one hand, a health officer had to resemble, to some extent, the itinerant circumcisers so that he would be perceived by locals as a legitimate circumciser to the extent necessary to break down the bonds between itinerant circumcisers and families. On the other hand, performing circumcision could mean losing professional prestige and being on a par with itinerant circumcisers. As a result, this new name allowed health officers to maintain a balance between cultivating familiarity with potential clients and maintaining their distinctiveness.

How did the ambivalence toward Sünnetçi play itself out on the ground? How did health officers/fenni sünnetçi seek to gain recognition while simultaneously creating their difference from itinerant circumcisers?

RECOGNITION

Summertime means the beginning of the time for circumcision. Meanwhile, modern techniques make this religiously required practice very easy. Thanks to these techniques, children get circumcised without pain. Moreover, they can play soccer or even go swimming a day after the circumcision. Kemal Özkan, the renowned circumciser in Turkey and the Middle East says: "Circumcision is now a science. I can perform it at any time of the year" (*Hürriyet*, June 2, 1976).

Mass publicity, mainly via newspapers like *Hürriyet*, was one strategy used by health officers to bring the new message of scientific circumcision ("circumcision is now a science") to the broader public during the developmentalist era. In addition to sporadically circulating ads marketing the service of painless circumcision, health officers used this platform as moral pioneers to educate the public about circumcision and to announce the benefits, such as safety and speedy recovery, of the surgical techniques. In continuity with the biopolitical and civilizational ethos of the post-Republic period, health officers joined other authorities, including representatives from the ministry of health, in warning families against unlicensed itinerant circumcisers, claiming that their lack of medical expertise could harm their sons. One health officer remarked in 1971:

For my job, I traveled to many places in Anatolia and I was horrified at seeing barbers who were performing circumcision in very bad conditions with the same straight razors that they were using to shave beards. This is a murder and must be stopped (*Hürriyet*, 1971).

The range of injuries nonmedical circumcisions could cause, it was claimed, included lifelong sexual dissatisfaction, sterility, urinary tract deformity, increased susceptibility to inflammation and sores, and psychological problems triggered by the aesthetics of a deformed penis (*Günaydın* 1972). Around the same time, news of circumcision-related malpractice and accidents began to appear in the public view: the story of a man who walked into a neighborhood, introduced himself as a circumciser, performed circumcisions, and then disappeared immediately after an operation that led to excessive bleeding; a report about a drunk circumciser who cut off too much of a boy's foreskin; cautionary tales of brothers who tried to circumcise each other or a boy who circumcised himself. These are just a few among the many news items that alarmingly made their way into the public imaginary, linking male circumcision with harm and risk.

Yet, the impact of printed media in garnering acceptance and visibility for medicalized circumcision remained limited, in part because itinerant circumcisers had served communities for generations and their longstanding relationships with boys' families became obstacles to health officers' efforts in making inroads into communities. Face-to-face dialogue was therefore another way for health officers to convince families of the benefits of surgical techniques. And families' reactions to health officers were not always pleasant.

Some families were unhappy with modern circumcision, as the new techniques changed the spatial and temporal organization of male circumcision. For example, the medicalized circumcision changed boys' bodily position during the operation. In the circumcisions performed by itinerant circumcisers, typically an apprentice or a male adult (an immediate family member or next of kin) would place the boy on his lap and put his arms around the boy's legs, keeping the legs wide and holding them as tightly as possible to prevent movement during the operation. By contrast, health officers had children lie down on a flat surface (the floor, a dinner table, an operating table, or a stretcher) so that the medical professionals could see better and more easily stitch the incisions. When they first began to perform circumcision, health officers said, a few families expressed discontent regarding this change. Some of my interviewees recounted that they continued to circumcise boys in the old position for a while and others mentioned that families were not usually "stubborn" about the boys' bodily position and would often let them proceed with the horizontal position.

The extended operation time drew sharper criticism from families than the change in physical position. Local anesthesia and sutures prolonged the operation, because health officers now had to wait for a few minutes before the anesthesia kicked in and needed extra time for stitching the incision after removing the foreskin. Some families, accustomed to the old circumcisions performed without local anesthesia and sutures, found the additional time tedious and unnecessary. Given that male circumcision was a painful operation, they believed that the operation should be completed as quickly as possible and valued dexterity and quickness as qualities in circumcisers. Some health officers reported that it was not uncommon to hear scornful remarks from families, such as "Old circumcisers would have finished it by now!" Fenni Sünnetçi Hüseyin—whose bitter remarks about families were mentioned in the previous section—recalled tension with families about speed:

AUTHOR: Did they [families] let you use local anesthesia?
HÜSEYIN: No! What have I been telling you? [he gets upset] I did not even try. They would beat me up if I did. We used to say, 'Look, your kid would not feel pain if we used it.' They would not listen to you. They would not give up on their customs. They used to say, "You are too slow! What kind of circumciser are you?" They were comparing us with barbers.

Similarly, health officers represented stitches as an important innovation in male circumcision, for its capacity to minimize possible complications (such as inflammation and infection) that an open incision might cause. Yet, some health officers found that families opposed suturing as well. Erkan, a health officer, had finished medical school in 1968, completed his compulsory military service afterward (during which he circumcised more than a hundred soldiers), and then received an additional year of training in the specialty of anesthesia. In 1974, Erkan was assigned to a state hospital in a small town in the Central Anatolia Region of Turkey and there he began to perform circumcision. He found himself competing against an itinerant circumciser with decades of experience and strong communal ties. When I asked Sünnetçi Erkan about families' reactions to the medical techniques, he replied:

ERKAN: Let me tell you. I was going to their houses to circumcise their children, and I was telling them I was going to use local anesthesia and sutures. Some of them objected: "What are you doing? Are you performing surgery? Why are you numbing it? Why are you suturing it?" I was saying: "Take it or leave it" [işinize gelirse]. Then they got used to it.
AUTHOR: Why did these families not want you to use local anesthesia and sutures in the beginning?
ERKAN: Well, in the past, barbers used to just cut off the foreskin with a straight razor and then leave. Maybe they were just putting powder on it. That would take two minutes or even one minute. In our method, you apply local anesthesia and wait for it to kick in, and then you suture the veins. It was taking eight or ten minutes. That bothered people.
AUTHOR: Were they telling you that you were too slow?
ERKAN: Yes, of course. I heard the question "Are you performing surgery?" many times. In some villages, conservative [tutucu] villages, they said, "Circumcision

is not a circumcision without blood." I was saying, "What does this have to do with blood? It is good there is no blood."

As in the case of local anesthesia, some families, at least initially, expressed doubts about the use of stitches, as it made the duration of the operation longer. Male circumcision tends to cause anxiety, not only for boys but also the other family members watching the operations, as boys often cry from fear, if not pain. I discuss this anxiety in depth in chapters 4 and 5, and it suffices here to say that it would not be too far-fetched to claim that the prolonged operation time in the 1960s exacerbated families' anxiety concerning the operation.

As Sünnetçi Erkan's words indicated, stitches could be seen as unacceptable for another reason. As in the ritual of sacrificing animals on Eid al-Adha, the symbolic gesture of releasing blood was for some families a necessary component of the circumcision ritual. These families' reactions toward the use of sutures could therefore be harsh sometimes: for instance, chasing away health officers who refused to honor their requests that the operation be performed without sutures. As one health officer recalled, "They initially insisted that I would not use stitches. I told them that I could make it bleed this way, too, but they did not let me use stitches." That said, the health officers I spoke with emphasized that families grew accustomed to the technique of stitching over time.

In the absence of consent for the use of the new techniques, some health officers, like Erkan, refused to perform those operations and left. Others made compromises, primarily because they did not want to lose customers. Accordingly, a couple of health officers I spoke to reported having initially used itinerant circumcisers' instruments. Günay, a sixty-two-year-old health officer, was one of those who used a straight razor to cut off the foreskin during the first few years of his practice. Sünnetçi Günay had completed his medical education in 1968 and was assigned to a town in northern Turkey: "There was no doctor in the town, and I was one of the few health professionals. We were kind of doctors." He then added:

My family was poor. My father was a shepherd. We were living in poverty. When I was assigned as a civil servant in 1968, I could take care of my mother and father. This job [civil service] gave me a lot. I now own a house and a store. I am popular here. I have circumcised many kids. Let me tell you what a doctor who was like a brother to me said to me once: "If you stay somewhere long enough, you can become popular there." Or let me put it this way: a brand.

When I asked him about the early years of his practice as a circumciser:

I performed circumcisions outside my regular working hours [as a civil servant]. I first used a straight razor. Using the straight razor was part of the practice at that time, and that's what people were accustomed to. There were [itinerant] circumcisers who received permission for performing circumcision. I don't know how, though. They had improved their skills by performing circumcision repeatedly. They were using straight razors. We fought against them. Not only them but also others like iğneci. Now those circumcisers are no longer performing circumcision.

"Iğneci" referred to female healers who administered injections within communities and, of all my interviewees, Sünnetçi Günay was the only health officer who had struggled against both these female healers and traditional circumcisers at the same time. Unlike other health officers, Sünnetçi Günay could not use his legal status against itinerant circumcisers, because the senior itinerant circumcisers of his area were among a very small percentage of itinerant circumcisers who had a license to perform the procedure. Thus, using a straight razor for operations was a way of making his practice more appealing to the locals while establishing himself as the community's circumciser.

Besides straight razors, a few health officers also used herbs at first. Fenni Sünnetçi Muharrem was born in 1946 in a small town in western Turkey. After completing elementary and middle school, he was able to register for medical school: "I was coming from a poor family. I wanted to go to a vocational school, instead of a regular high school, so that I could begin to make a living [hayata atılmak] sooner than later." Before settling into his current situation in 1975 in a city of the Central Anatolia Region, he had been assigned to two separate cities, where he had circumcised only a few boys. When he wanted to perform circumcision more regularly at his current location, he realized that doing so would not be easy:

AUTHOR: Were there other circumcisers when you began to perform circumcision here?

MUHARREM: Yes, there were a few people who also finished medical school and came here before me. Two of them were my classmates. There was a senior health officer, and I observed him performing circumcisions a lot. There were also Abdals.

AUTHOR: Did you have any interaction with them?

MUHARREM: No, but I started going to the neighborhoods wherein they performed circumcisions. They were telling people that local anesthesia and stitches would emasculate boys [erkekliği öldürüyor].

AUTHOR: But there was no tension between you and them?

MUHARREM: Well, kind of. Once, I was performing a circumcision and this Abdal was watching me. He himself was not a circumciser, but apparently his dad used to be. Their techniques were different. They were using a straight razor and then putting some powder on it [the incision]. As I was circumcising the kid, he [the Abdal] said, "My dad would have circumcised four or five kids by now." Then I replied, "Well, your dad should do it then!" But this was a minor tension. It did not really last long.

AUTHOR: What about families? Did they like stitches?

MUHARREM: No, it took a while, three or five years, before they got used to it. You know, as a nation, we are not open to innovation. We first must see the result, then we accept the innovation.

AUTHOR: What sort of reactions did you get?

MUHARREM: Some families insisted I use old techniques, and I sometimes complied with them so that I would not lose customers. But once the requests for old techniques increased too much, I started saying no. I used to say, "Look, I am working only on the foreskin, not the penis. Nothing should happen to the penis."

AUTHOR: What sort of old techniques did you use? Straight razor and herbs?

MUHARREM: No, I did not use the straight razor, but I used herbs a couple of times instead of sutures. Once I switched to sutures, some families got upset. There was one family who insisted on seeing blood, and when I rejected them, they just left.

Families became upset about Sünnetçi Muharrem's style, partly because his circumcisions were taking longer than the traditional circumcisions and partly because they believed the medical techniques to be either too invasive and potentially damaging to penises or incompatible with their beliefs about the symbolic value of the blood in male circumcision. And Sünnetçi Muharrem's temporary acquiescence to families' demands should be seen in light of the fact that he as a young health officer competed against not only itinerant circumcisers but also health officers. Like Sünnetçi Günay, Sünnetçi Muharrem also briefly used a nonsurgical technique to gain a footing within the competitive field of male circumcision. He intentionally blurred the boundary between itinerant circumcisers and himself.

Sünnetçi Muharrem was not the only health officer disturbed by the association between infertility or emasculation and their medical techniques. Health officer Selami began to perform circumcision in 1983 in a northwestern city, where he had moved after finishing his medical education in 1973. He worked at a hospital until his retirement. He was one of the few circumcisers who requested I use their real names. "Are you going to translate your book to Turkish? I want to read it!" he said. He also prided himself on fighting what he considered misconceptions around medical circumcision techniques:

SELAMİ: I am the one who popularized fenni sünnet [scientific circumcision] here. I was using local anesthesia, sutures, scalpel, forceps, everything. I was the one who was performing the kind of circumcisions that professors were doing at hospitals. First, families did not want the needle [local anesthesia]. They used to say, "No, not with the needle. It causes infertility."

AUTHOR: Sorry, what?

SELAMİ: Infertility. That was the rumor among people. I said, "Look, this is how I am doing it." Some families got mad at me.

AUTHOR: How long did it take for people to get used to it?

SELAMİ: Five years, ten years. You know, with television and the internet, people are enlightened now [bilinçli]. I was telling families, "Look, when you scratch your arm, nothing happens to your arm, right? Only your skin, right? When you go to a dentist, they also numb you. It is the same thing."

As a moral pioneer, Sünnetçi Selami viewed his efforts as part of educating peasants about modern medicine and dispelling the rumors about the new techniques. He and some of the other health officers interpreted families' distrust in these techniques as a matter of ignorance and resistance to change. Yet, it never occurred to them that their presence as state actors, and not their medical techniques per se, could account for at least some of the distrust. As chapter 1 shows, most of the itinerant circumcisers received no negative reaction from families about the use of the medical circumcision techniques, as these circumcisers had been known by the families for generations.

Another strategy that young health officers deployed to gain locals' acceptance was to forge contractual relationships with senior circumcisers, a strategy that proved beneficial for two main reasons. First, it helped young practitioners improve their circumcision skills. Most of the health officers I interviewed mentioned the lack of rigorous training in circumcision in medical schools, which at first undermined their self-confidence as circumcisers. Some of my interviewees waited before beginning to perform circumcision, rather than starting immediately after completing (high school–level) vocational medical school, due to their worries about making mistakes and consequently failing to gain families' trust. One way to address this problem was to observe and learn from senior and experienced circumcisers, whether they were health officers themselves or even itinerant circumcisers. Thus, when Fenni Sünnetçi Bünyamin wanted to start his circumcision practice at the age of thirty-two, he received informal training from a senior health officer. Like other health officers, Bünyamin's exposure to the practice of circumcision had been minimal during his education:

AUTHOR: Can you tell me a little bit about your education?

BÜNYAMİN: It was both theoretical and practical. I took all kinds of courses: mathematics, geometry, literature, physics, anatomy, music, biology, military, and public health.

AUTHOR: What about practical training?

BÜNYAMİN: Some senior nurses taught me how to administer an injection, dress wounds, etc. Since the nurses taught us how to do it, when I got sick, I gave myself shots.

AUTHOR: What about circumcision?

BÜNYAMİN: There was a doctor who visited our anatomy class once. He drew a penis on the blackboard and showed how to measure and cut it off, and told us all the details. In that class, I got curious and decided I was going to do this job after graduation.

AUTHOR: So you did not practice male circumcision at school, then, right?

BÜNYAMİN: No.

AUTHOR: And did you start performing circumcision right after graduation?

BÜNYAMİN: No, I did not think I was ready. This is a stressful job. You are working on a precious organ, and if you make a mistake, you can ruin the boy's life.

AUTHOR: When did you start, then?

BÜNYAMİN: I came here [a town in southern Turkey] and worked as an assistant for a circumciser for two years.

AUTHOR: Was he a health officer, too?

BÜNYAMİN: Yes, he was. He is no longer alive. It was a master-apprentice relationship.

AUTHOR: How did you help him?

BÜNYAMİN: He let me administer injections, and I was also preparing the bandage that he used to dress the incision. I observed him. That's how I learned.

AUTHOR: Did he observe your first circumcision?

BÜNYAMİN: No, he did not. For my first circumcision, there was a family who wanted to have their son circumcised but did not have money. No one would circumcise him for free. But I did. This is how I started.

Sünnetçi Bünyamin at first did not want to perform circumcision, as he found the job too stressful. The phrase "precious organ" frequently came up in my conversations with circumcisers, including itinerant circumcisers. The phrase reveals the emotional pressure around the ethic of care, the too-muchness associated with performing circumcision—the pressure that circumcisers have confronted in various ways.

Moreover, as chapter 3 shows, circumcising poor boys was a common training method for young and inexperienced health officers who, like Sünnetçi Bünyamin, wanted to improve their circumcision skills in a short period. Unlike some of the other cases, Sünnetçi Bünyamin did not have to worry about competing against health officers and was able to gain support from a senior health officer, mainly because of the high demand for circumcision in his area and the fact that his master was close to retirement (circumcisers typically retired in their late sixties). His informal relationship with the senior circumciser enabled him to gain the practical knowledge missing from his medical education.

Those health officers trained by senior health officers spoke openly with me about these temporary arrangements. Health officers were, however, unwilling to talk about the same arrangements when the informal training had been provided by itinerant circumcisers. Most of them mentioned these associations only in passing, without going into further details (though itinerant circumcisers separately helped me fill in the blanks). Arguably, more thorough expositions of these arrangements would destabilize the idealized self-image health officers aimed to sustain not only in their dialogues with me but also in their practices—a self-image shaped by a sense of superiority over itinerant circumcisers.

Gazanfer, now age eighty-one, was the only health officer who was upfront about these otherwise embarrassing arrangements. Having completed his medical education at a medical school (sağlık koleji) in the 1950s, Sünnetçi Gazanfer was just beginning to perform circumcision in a western city of Turkey when he received training from an itinerant circumciser:

GAZANFER: We studied it theoretically, but not practically. We were forty, fifty students, and we just watched a doctor circumcising one or two kids. Sure, it was not enough, but after watching him I decided that was what I wanted to do.

AUTHOR: So you did not perform any circumcision on your own?

GAZANFER: No, and when I came here, there was no health officer and only one guy who was circumcising everyone.

AUTHOR: Was he a barber?

GAZANFER: No, but his master was a barber. He learned it from him. He was not sağlıkçı [health professional]. He liked raki and, say, you called him for circumcision for your kids, he would say to you: "Make chicken and serve me a bottle of raki." This was how he negotiated with families for compensation.

One day, I ran into him at this tavern in a nearby town. I was a regular and had befriended the owner of the tavern. I sent to his [the itinerant circumciser's] table a bottle of raki. He got upset and asked who I was. His friends said, "Health officer Gazanfer." He then said, "What is wrong with that guy? I do not know him. Take this back!" But I did not give up, and another night, I sent him a fruit assortment of banana, orange, apple, etc. He liked that. He then asked the owner to introduce him to me. I went up to his table. I told him, "Look, you are a master [usta], and I am very eager to learn it." He replied, "Kid, I like you. I could teach you to perform circumcision, but that would harm me. Circumcision is my means of livelihood. How would I know that you would not turn up as a competitor?" I said to him that I would not perform it in his territory. I made a promise and kept it. He then said, "I have to teach you [to prepare] the powder."

AUTHOR: Powder?

GAZANFER: Yes, powder. I said, "No, I am a health officer, and I will get my stuff from a pharmacy. I use cream, ointment." Later, I found out how he prepared his powder. He was using gallnut . . . and used to grind it on a mortar and pestle and then add something else but I cannot remember what it was. He was worried about bleeding.

AUTHOR: This was for post-operation, right?

GAZANFER: Yes, but since we were technical, we knew which veins would bleed, and we would stitch them. If we were too busy and did not have enough time, we would dress the incision. He and I went to a few villages, and he taught me how to cut the foreskin off. He even let me do it. Then I started getting calls for circumcision.

AUTHOR: How old were you when you performed your first circumcision?

GAZANFER: Twenty-one.

Gazanfer set his mind on becoming a circumciser after having watched a couple of circumcisions during his education. Following his graduation, as a young and ambitious health officer, Gazanfer saw a window of opportunity to realize his dream in his new locale, which had only one circumciser. Yet, he was also cautious about starting his own practice prematurely, given that his medical education hadn't prepared him for such a major and risky undertaking. Once the possibility of a future threat was avoided, Sünnetçi Gazanfer's mentor agreed to help him, out of kindness and without expecting any material benefit in return. Sünnetçi Gazanfer's insistence on informally improving his skills eventually paid off: the senior itinerant circumciser retired, and Gazanfer expanded his practice and became the most popular circumciser in the area.

As discussed in chapter 1, not all itinerant circumcisers were willing to train young health officers without expecting anything in return, as some of them needed legal protection. Health officer Emek offered an unlicensed senior itinerant circumciser such a safeguard in exchange for training in male circumcision. Emek completed medical school in 1963 and was later assigned to a town in a city of the Central Anatolia Region. When we met, he first took me to a nearby village, where I interviewed an itinerant circumciser. Then, he and I sat down for a conversation about his own practice:

AUTHOR: How did you learn to perform circumcision?

EMEK: They only showed us once at school. We all watched a doctor circumcising a couple of kids. I did not practice it at school.

AUTHOR: What about after you came here?

EMEK: There was only one circumciser in town X at that time. He said, "I do not have a diploma. Come with me and you can learn it."

AUTHOR: So he was not a health officer, right?

EMEK: No. He had learned it from his father. I tagged along with him. If he was asked about his license by police, he was going to use me as a shield.

AUTHOR: How did your first circumcision go?

EMEK: One day he turned to me and said, "Okay, you have been watching me for a long while now. You are ready." I was, of course, very nervous. But I think it went well.

Credentials, which authorize their holders to perform certain tasks attached to certain positions, institute a powerful, and yet ultimately artificial, dividing line separating one group of people from another group (or groups). Sociologists highlight that credentials carry more symbolic than practical significance. Skills are largely learned on the job instead of during education (Collins 2019). Sünnetçi Emek's lack of experience in male circumcision left him ill-equipped for the reality of the community into which he graduated. For health officers like Sünnetçi Emek, their sense of professional worth was undermined, if not eroded altogether, by a sense of inadequacy regarding their skills in postgraduate life—a shortcoming that they tried to amend by making temporary arrangements with senior circumcisers. With this strategy, they further accumulated cultural capital in the form of skills and avoided making mistakes that would harm both boys and the reputation they diligently sought to foster as circumcisers.

Some health officers used the same cooperative strategy to overcome their position as strangers within their new communities. A rationale behind the Turkish state's centralized appointment system for civil servants was that it prevented unofficial preexisting bonds with the local foci of authority from interfering with the officers' civilizing mission. Throughout the history of the Republic, the centralized bureaucratic system of surveillance tended to generate suspicion and distrust on both sides (civil servants as well as peasants), as the system was "informed by a particular view of peasants, namely that they are conservative, uninterested in change and unintelligent. They must be led rather than being included as partners, and the trained outsider is sent in as the leader, the agent of change . . ." (Delaney 1991, p. 220). In the case of male circumcision, to wrest control of circumcision away from the itinerant circumcisers health officers had to create bonds with communities, build trust, and accumulate social capital in the form of social networks and group membership.

Paradoxically, one way to achieve this goal was to gain access to the itinerant circumcisers' networks. Barber Sezai, an itinerant circumciser, helped health officers connect with families who otherwise would have had their sons circumcised by itinerant circumcisers. At the age of seventeen, Barber Sezai had learned to perform circumcision from his master, who was also a barber, and then Sezai began to go to circumcisions with health officers in the early 1960s:

AUTHOR: Why did health officers want to bring you along?

SEZAİ: I am a tradesman and I knew many people. I told them I could find them customers only if they let me come with them. I worked with two health officers. Obviously, not all health officers were good practitioners. Before I met health officers, I used to perform circumcision without local anesthesia. Then I watched how they worked. I observed old [traditional] circumcisers as well, but they did not know how to stop the bleeding.

AUTHOR: What did the arrangements involve exactly?

SEZAİ: I did not have a license, and if the police came, health officers stepped in and told them that they were the ones who were performing the circumcisions.

AUTHOR: What about the fee?

SEZAİ: We split it. We did this only a few times though. Then we parted ways.

It is one thing to start your practice at a new place without preexisting social connections, but it is another and much more difficult thing to make a name as a stranger who introduces techniques and skills unfamiliar to a community. Young health officers wanted to overcome this barrier by taking advantage of the trust that Barber Sezai had among locals. Barbershops are, as we saw in the previous chapter, crucial settings for establishing connections among men in Turkey. Barbers engage in daily conversations with their regular customers about a wide range of topics, including soccer games and politics, and develop personal relations with them. As a respected long-term member of the community, Barber Sezai was thus well positioned to vouch for the health officers and their medical techniques.

Not all health officers encountered difficulties in starting practices in their new communities. When they did, such strategies as persuasion, compromise, and cooperation enabled them to stake their claims regarding medical circumcision and better articulate the benefits of their techniques to the public, as well as to remedy their status as outsiders. In doing so, they made themselves into circumcisers who were not only legal but also legitimate in the eyes of families, and they medicalized the practice.

A prevailing theory of medicalization suggests that medicalization typically moves a family and community-centered event or practice (for instance, childbirth) to a medical setting within the control of medical professionals, disempowering local actors (for instance, midwives) (Cosminsky 2016; Duden 1993; Ehrenreich and English 2010). However, the medicalization of male circumcision in the 1960s in Turkey, as we have seen, did not follow the same trajectory. Although, in theory, families could have their sons circumcised in medical settings, this rarely occurred, and the operation remained embedded within communities. The persistence of the communal nature of the operation was aligned with health officers' wish to keep their practices unrecorded and untaxed. As we will see in the second part of this book, the separation between the home and communal network and the circumcision operation did not begin until the late 1990s and early 2000s.

PARTIAL IMITATIONS

This chapter has paid close attention to the complex identifications taking place between health officers and itinerant circumcisers—identifications comparable to those between colonizers and colonized. Using a Lacanian psychoanalytical framework, sociologist George Steinmetz (2007) and critical theorist Homi Bhabha (1994) examine the ambiguous cross-identifications between colonizers and colonized in German and Indian contexts, respectively. While the former shows how the colonizers' partial identification with the colonized was essential to the colonial governance, the latter draws attention to how the colonized are encouraged to become similar to, but not exactly the same as, the colonizers. This is so because the full imitation of the colonizer would undermine the colonizer's strategy of governance based on cultural differences. Steinmetz and Bhabha show that the subjectivities of both colonizers and colonized are ambivalent and contradictory, as they are based on a play of sameness and difference vis-à-vis each other.

A similar play can also be observed in our case where itinerant circumcisers and health officers imitate each other. The Turkish state's strategy of usurpation aiming to dispossess itinerant circumcisers prepared the ground for health officers' ambivalent attachments to medicalization. To establish themselves in their new communities, health officers as state agents sought to imitate their rivals, but only in a partial way. Like itinerant circumcisers, they went to families' homes for circumcisions. Although the ministry of health assigned health officers to specific workplaces and regular schedules, they followed the itinerant circumcisers' work model and schedule and visited private homes in cities, towns, and villages mostly on the weekends to circumcise boys at homes in informal fee-for-service arrangements. Yet, given that itinerant circumcisers were stigmatized in the modern and national imagination of Turkey, health officers also carefully and anxiously differentiated themselves from itinerant circumcisers by introducing medical techniques and invoking scientific discourses and a medical ethos. Fenni Sünnetçi thus represented a compromised professional identity fundamental to the reorganization of male circumcision under the medical authority in Turkey.

Health officers sustained their desires for medicalization by integrating what they otherwise disavowed: Sünnetçi. Sünnetçi was an object of both attraction and repulsion, which made health officers prone to such emotions as anger, resentment, and bitterness, especially when they felt like they were mistaken for itinerant circumcisers by families (or the author). Attachment always carries the possibility of becoming lost in the Other while seeking to bring the Other closer. Fenni Sünnetçi was therefore both defensive and transformative, simultaneously affirming professional prestige and reminding health officers of a (possibly embarrassing) resemblance. It was almost the same as Sünnetçi, but not quite.

From the outset, the medicalization of male circumcision in Turkey was characterized by a series of tensions. Health officers not only aimed at shaping the demands for male circumcision by transforming families' habitus into a medical one but also sought to channel that demand toward themselves as the sole legal practitioners. However, unlike more sophisticated medical tasks, medicalized male circumcision, as shown in chapter 1, could be learned, imitated, and reappropriated. Thus, while health officers were keen to maintain their distinction from itinerant circumcisers stigmatized in their eyes, itinerant circumcisers' adoption of medical expertise made their fear come true.

As we shall examine later in the book, this blurring in identity has recently served as an ideological ground for doctors and hospitals to appropriate male circumcision from health officers. Yet, the full understanding of this ideological transformation requires an examination of another form of circumcision: mass circumcisions. This is so because the ways health officers performed mass operations during the developmentalist era rendered them a target for criticism that has placed health officers and itinerant circumcisers in the same stigmatized category of sünnetçi. The next chapter turns to these charity-based circumcisions.

3 | MASS CIRCUMCISION

I talked to Sünnetçi Muhsin in a small town on the north coast of the Marmara Sea. Sünnetçi Muhsin graduated from medical school (sağlık koleji) in Istanbul in 1966 and had been performing circumcision for forty-two years. During his education, he observed a few operations performed under general anesthesia by doctors using scissors. "Mine is practical, though," Sünnetçi Muhsin said, referring to his preference for a scalpel and local anesthesia. With general anesthesia and scissors, he emphasized, an operation takes forty-five minutes or even an hour. "They were removing the foreskin in pieces with scissors. That was not practical," he added. During the developmentalist era, doctors performed circumcision mostly for training purposes, without feeling pressured to turn it into a routine business activity. For Sünnetçi Muhsin, the operation had to be both fast and safe so that he could efficiently compete. He thus later learned the faster method informally from another doctor after graduation.

I introduced myself to Sünnetçi Muhsin right before his noon prayer, and he agreed to talk to me at a café near the mosque afterward:

AUTHOR: Why did you want to start doing this in the first place?
MUHSİN: To be honest, for economic reasons.
AUTHOR: Was it appealing?
MUHSİN: Yes, it was. But you know, there are poor people [fakir fukara] in villages. We don't charge them anything. It is not easy to become firmly established in this profession [bu meslekte tutunmak kolay değil]. You shouldn't give heed to material things [maddiyata önem vermeyeceksin]. For this job, first, you should be skillful, and second, you need to be social [çenen kuvvetli olacak]. People should like you. If possible, you should make an appearance in newspapers or even on TV. You can be famous, then.
AUTHOR: So, self-marketing is important.
MUHSİN: It is. You can't do much without that.
AUTHOR: Were you ever in a newspaper?

78

MUHSİN: Yes, I was. They took a photo of me at a mass circumcision festival. People know me here. Of course, people would not know me in another city. But they do know me here.

A striking aspect of my interview with Sünnetçi Muhsin was his ambivalent sentiments regarding his economic motives for performing circumcision. On the one hand, he highlighted economic calculation as the main driver behind his decision to perform circumcision. On the other hand, he at times downplayed its importance. His account oscillated between the pursuit and maximization of personal gain and maintaining an altruistic self- and public image—an image crafted for himself and locals as well as the researcher.

Circumcisers, especially health officers, consistently told me: "We are not in this for money. This is a matter of health." They dodged my questions about circumcision service prices and at the same time alluded to economic incentives in performing circumcision. They often condemned other practitioners for violating another moral principle of the field: altruism. If one principle has been "do not harm," the other one was/is altruism—an imperative that medical tasks should be performed without being corrupted by profit-seeking motives. They imputed such motives to others while representing themselves as selfless practitioners. In doing so, I argue, they attached themselves ambivalently to the rational, calculative, and self-interested subject position by distancing themselves from it.

As we saw in the previous chapters, health officers gained control over male circumcision by introducing medical expertise starting in the 1960s. To accomplish this, they had to manage the tension between professional prestige and wider popular acceptance. Focusing on the same medicalization process during the same historical period, this chapter primarily turns to another status-related tension, one between self-interest and altruism, a commitment to others' well-being. Altruism is key to medical professionals' habitus, as health professionals are expected to put their patients' interests above their own (Timmermans and Hyeyoung 2010). Although the meanings of "self-interest" and "public good" depend on cultural contexts, power relations, and collective struggles, "a normative orientation grounded in the community" (Gorman and Sandefur 2011, p. 278) remains woven into the raison d'être of medical professions in general.

In what follows, I examine how circumcisers managed the contradiction between self-interest and altruism in male circumcision. Health officers' challenge to itinerant circumcisers in the 1960s heightened the competition between practitioners on an unprecedented scale, further monetized circumcision services, and strengthened calculative reasoning in the field—changes that ran the risk of coming into conflict with practitioners' altruistic self-perception and public image. Accordingly, the chapter claims that mass circumcisions organized for low-income families, where hundreds of boys get circumcised on the same day, enabled practitioners, particularly health officers, to sustain their altruism and thus their profit-seeking dispositions. Pursuing profits would be, health officers felt, frowned upon by their communities, which made it impossible for them to perform or internalize the position in a straightforward manner. They rather bound themselves to the position only indirectly and ambivalently through a kind of reprieve from its prescriptions by performing mass circumcisions.

Mass circumcisions rest upon the perpetual production of the distinction and hierarchy between the poor and nonpoor via policies and informal and formal mechanisms and procedures that aim to manage, rather than eradicate, poverty. In this chapter, I trace mass circumcisions' changing role in legitimizing rule, power, and status from the Ottoman Era until the end of the developmentalist era. While mass circumcisions in the late Ottoman period enabled the rulers to disavow their *political* interests, the charity organizations involved gained an additional significance starting in the 1960s: the disavowal of *economic* interest.[1] Medicalized mass circumcisions during the developmentalist era transformed low-income families into anonymous bodies of spectacle, thereby enabling circumcisers to disavow their economic interests and fashion themselves as carers of the poor.

The chapter also shows that mass circumcisions proved to be a crucial opportunity for young health officers to develop their skills and accumulate cultural capital. As the previous chapters point out, newly graduated health officers lacked experience in performing circumcision, putting them at a disadvantage compared to senior circumcisers. To redress this imbalance, health officers engaged in various strategies such as short-term arrangements with senior circumcisers. Performing mass circumcision was another strategy used by health officers, who could circumcise large numbers of boys in very short periods of time at these gatherings.

That said, circumcisers' relationship with mass circumcisions and the benevolent self was far from straightforward, as these operations also inadvertently generated a moral contradiction for them. The last section of the chapter highlights the tenuous relationship between the promise of medicalization and mass circumcisions during the developmentalist era, as the operations were characterized by unhygienic venues, multiple uses of the same instruments, unstitched incisions, and fast cuttings—a level of care that fell below the standards practitioners cherished as good and desirable at that time. Consequently, health officers' guilt over mass circumcision—the unnerving feeling captured by their renaming of mass circumcisions as "mass massacres"—motivated some of them to make changes to the organization of mass circumcision in order to solve the class-based inequalities in male circumcision.

Framing practitioners' participation in mass circumcision charity events in terms of their interest in maximizing their power should not be taken to present a cynical view that assumes an ulterior self-serving motive camouflaged by an altruistic façade. I do not intend to speculate about, let alone cast a suspicious glance on, circumcisers' intentions and honesty. Instead, my point is simple: circumcisers' pragmatic attitude toward mass circumcisions was socially produced, in the sense that, together, the competitive circumcision field and the welfare governance characterized by the state's neglect of low-income families induced circumcisers to instrumentalize mass circumcisions. Participating in mass circumcision events acted as an imperative: circumcisers often performed these operations, as my interviewees said, because otherwise others would do it. And this instrumentalization caused an emotional burden for them. My analysis focuses on the organizational infrastructure of mass circumcision and its symbolic and affective significance for circumcisers, rather than their intentions.

IMPERIAL CIRCUMCISION FESTIVALS

During the Ottoman Empire period, sultans organized imperial circumcision festivals for princes as a public platform for displaying royal power and sending messages to Ottoman subjects and foreign powers. While until the mid-fifteenth century dynastic marriages were the major public celebrations, afterward circumcision festivals replaced wedding ceremonies in importance as concubinage replaced marriage in the Ottoman Empire (Topal 2020). The general themes of these meticulously crafted and elaborate events included imperial grandeur, justice, and royal dedication to the tradition of the Prophet (Terzioglu 1995). The events could take as long as fifty-five days—as did, for instance, the 1582 festival—during which time sultans engaged in various performative acts: paying the debts of debtors and having them released from prison, expressing world dominion by exhibiting exotic animals like elephants and giraffes as well as performers from all around the world, and punishing artisans who violated market regulations (Rahimi 2014). The imperial circumcision festivals included different entertainment activities such as ceremonial reception, musical performances, communal feasts, athletic games, mock battles on castles, and firework displays (Rahimi 2014).

These festivals enabled social groups to relay messages to the sultan and the public, messages reflecting changing power dynamics within and beyond the state. In 1582, for instance, artisan processions were introduced into imperial ceremonies, epitomizing urban guilds' growing social and economic power and their mediating role between the artisans and the state in the Ottoman society (Terzioglu 1995). More than a hundred and fifty guilds engaged in spectacles demonstrating their skills and merits in front of Sultan Murat III (r. 1574–1595). The sultan enjoyed the rivalry between "different guilds as each association tried to make their procession more spectacular as they vied for greater public admiration" (Rahimi 2014, p. 98).

The circumcision of a young prince as the future sultan and the attendant celebrations contributed to fashioning the sultan's sacred body with symbols of virility, prowess, and fertility. The symbolic meaning of imperial circumcisions was evident in the use of the nahil, the central ritual object of imperial circumcision ceremonies, "a large pyramid-shaped wooden pole laden either with real or artificial flowers or with edible objects like fruit or sweets" (Rahimi 2014, p. 100). The nahil represented birth, male strength, fertility, and generation as well as the sultan's power and authority. The ritual procession involved a series of communal preparations for "taking the young prince away from the world of women and introducing him to the outer world of the public" as a site of royal strength and political power (Rahimi 2014, p. 105). Accordingly, the nahil is first kept in the maternal domain of the young prince's mother (valide sultan) at the Old Palace and is then taken to "an outer world (city spaces), as the wooden poles are paraded in the streets outside of the palace " (Rahimi 2014, p. 105). The nahil then returns to the palace where the processions began. The series of events was meant to dramatize the young prince's passage toward manhood, which required his separation from his mother.

Another conspicuous feature of imperial circumcisions was that the circumcision of poor and nonpoor boys took place as parts of the same events. During the circumcision festival organized by Sultan Murat III for his son Prince Mehmed, between three thousand and ten thousand boys of poor families were circumcised alongside Prince Mehmed. Surgeons first circumcised several boys every day, and then the chief surgeon circumcised the prince in a special room at the end of the festival. The sultan also gave small gifts to the boys upon the completion of circumcisions (Sari et al. 1996). Poor boys' circumcisions provided an opportunity for the sultan to instrumentalize generosity as a technique of legitimacy and to foster solidarity and union between himself and his subjects (Özbek 2008). He displayed his altruistic intentions, signaling that he and his son were one of them. Put differently, the sultan, via mass circumcision, disavowed his political motives and gains.

As scarce as our knowledge of the techniques that surgeons used at imperial circumcisions is, one Ottoman surgeon, Şerafeddin Sabuncuoğlu, explains his techniques in detail in his book titled *Cerrahiyye-i Ilhaniye* (Royal Surgery), which was published in 1465. Sabuncuoğlu describes special scissors with slightly curved blade tips. He applied wads and dressings and then ashes of dried gourds or fine white flour for the incisions. For wound treatment, "egg yolk cooked in rose water and ground with the oil of roses was applied and kept on until the following day. The wound was then dressed with other medicaments until it healed" (Sari et al. 1996, p. 923). Sabuncuoğlu's book also recommends double ligations for healthy and safe circumcisions.

Throughout the nineteenth century, male circumcision became woven into the Ottoman state's purposes of centralization and modernization. Especially during the reign of Sultan Abdulhamid II (1842–1918), the Ottoman state associated religious piety with political loyalty, seeking to spread orthodox Sunnism among "those who did not strictly observe Islamic principles or perform the rituals" (Topal 2020, 3). Accordingly, the state initiated a campaign of circumcision and sent circumcisers to provinces distant from the capital to demarcate religious boundaries, thereby protecting Muslims against missionary influence (Topal 2020). Such campaigns were also an important opportunity for the Ottoman state to surveil the population. Whereas population surveys designed for conscription and tax purposes were met with population resistance, ranging from evasion to revolts, families were willing to welcome state-sponsored male circumcision to avoid its financial burden, which enabled the state to register the children (Topal 2020).

During the same period, male circumcision also became part of state-organized violence against non-Muslims. In 1891, the sultan established "The Hamidiye regiments," which were composed of Sunni Kurdish tribal and irregular groups, a well-armed force that would commit massacres against Armenians in the mid-1890s. As part of the anti-Christian violence, foreskin inspections became a common practice in mixed Muslim-Armenian settlements. Some Armenian clerics were targeted for circumcision to bring them into disrepute in the eyes of their communities. Also, "large numbers of Armenian men converted to Islam and were circumcised literally at the edge of the sword" (Sengul 2014, p. 37). In doing so, the sultan sought to establish Sunnism as the sine qua non of belonging and political loyalty in the Empire.

Furthermore, also under the rule of Sultan Abdulhamid II, imperial circumcisions underwent a critical transformation as well. By the end of the nineteenth century, as historian Nadir Özbek (2008) shows, various modern welfare institutions in the fields of public health, child welfare, and poverty relief had already begun to shape Ottoman subjects' lives. The sultan's welfare institutions were intended to "project an image of imperial paternalism, an image of a concerned monarchical father, foster public approval and popular legitimacy" (Özbek 2008, p. 44). The sultan viewed medical institutions as symbols of progress and science whereby he represented the Ottoman Empire as a modern state for the view of foreign powers.

As part of the new medical and scientific ethos, imperial circumcisions became medicalized. Hospitals began to carry out the operations on a mass scale, with surgical techniques glorified as a way of eliminating boys' pain and their families' concern regarding the operation. The sultan appointed prominent Ottoman surgeons to deliver scientifically informed procedures, and the medical institutions provided needy families with lunch and dinner and kept the circumcised boys overnight for follow-up evaluations. For circumcision events, state officials organized entertainment for families and gave children new shoes, clothes, and toys as gifts. The newspapers widely advertised these events, boasted about the number of circumcisions that were performed, and portrayed the sultan as a fatherly figure relieving the pain of the poor and bringing them happiness. As a result, medicalized imperial circumcisions created a public spectacle whereby the sultan crafted an image of a paternal figure who "was not only caring for his poor subjects, but he was providing them the best services the science and technology of the time enable[d] him to" (Özbek 2008, p. 44)—an effort consistent with the sultan's overall modernization policies as a new basis of legitimacy and rule.

During the Turkish War of Independence (1919–1923), the imperial family was deposed from power and the sultanate was abolished, with the declaration of the Republic of Turkey in 1923 driving the final nail into the coffin of the monarchy. And from the 1920s onwards, mass circumcisions underwent a series of transmutations that detached the symbolic and affective significance of these events from the sovereign's sublime body, transforming it into a stake among political and economic actors within a secular and democratic system—actors who now vied for their shares of the original sovereign benevolence associated with mass circumcisions. Furthermore, as male circumcision was commodified, the disavowal of political interest via the pious activity of charity, the main characteristic of (medicalized) mass circumcisions in the Ottoman Empire, has been supplemented by another one: the disavowal of economic interest.

This chapter and chapter 5 explain the changes in the meanings, functions, and organizations of mass circumcisions in detail. Chapter 5 traces political parties' and hospitals' involvement in mass circumcisions in the neoliberal era, and the rest of this chapter discusses how and why circumcisers participated in the network of mass circumcisions funded by civil society organizations during the developmentalist era. To answer these questions, however, it is necessary

first to examine the transformation of the Turkish welfare governance that addressed social security and poverty, and the inculcation of calculative reasoning
in the field of male circumcision—a combined development that potentially
conflicted with medical professionals' altruistic self- and public image.

POVERTY AND WELFARE IN TURKEY

In the pre–World War II single-party period, voluntary and philanthropic
associations represented the key agents in fighting against poverty in Turkey.
Affluent citizens, rather than the state, assumed responsibility in the realm of
social assistance. The three most significant social service institutions, Kızılay,
Society for the Protection of Children (later Cocuk Esirgeme Kurumu), and
the Association of Philanthropists (Yardım Sevenler Derneği), utilized a very
small share of the government budget and mostly relied on donations (Bugra
2007). As chapter 2 discusses, after the establishment of the Republic, the
Turkish elites faced the problems of a war-torn country where the majority of
the population lived in the countryside. In addition to the wars, villages in the
Central Anatolian plain were also drastically affected by the 1928 drought, and
the damage was only exacerbated by the Great Depression. The combination of
weak state initiatives and natural and human-made disasters during the early
decades of the Republic contributed greatly to rural poverty.

Despite the harsh social and economic conditions, rural-to-urban migration remained very low, mainly because the ruling elites concerned themselves
merely with preventing "abject poverty in the countryside from spreading to
the urban setting" (Bugra 2007, p. 39). They aimed to guarantee the survival of
peasant agriculture and small farmers by eliminating in 1925 the agricultural
tithe called aşar (a type of tax applied to agricultural output), thereby averting
the emergence of large agricultural production units and a consequent expansion of the displaced and dispossessed rural proletariat. These state policies
helped keep the flow of rural-urban migration in check until the 1960s.

As in many other parts of the world, in Turkey the end of World War II
marked the beginning of a new era in state-society relations, including institutional approaches to welfare. The gradual development of a formal social policy
and a new social security system involved "the provision of state-provided free
education at primary, secondary, and tertiary levels, and a combined public
health and pension system associated with employment status" (Buğra and
Keyder 2006, p. 213). Three public insurance schemes emerged (without a private insurance option): the Social Insurance Institution for Formal Workers in
1945, the Retirement Chest for Civil Servants in 1949, and the Pension Fund
for the Self-Employed in 1971. This eclectic welfare arrangement generated

two major forms of inequalities. One form was rooted within the insured population. The occupational groups covered by the public insurance schemes were ranked from top to bottom as civil servants, formal workers, and the self-employed according to the following criteria: premium rates, benefits, and the quality of the services provided for the beneficiaries. Civil servants, including health officers, made up the most privileged group, as they benefited from better benefits packages and higher quality of healthcare services than the other groups.

The other form of inequality divided the insured and the uninsured. The inegalitarian corporatist nature of the system protected only those in the formal sector, excluding the rural population and those employed in the urban informal sector. No health insurance scheme for the poor existed until 1992 (which I discuss in chapter 5). The ratio of the insured population covered by health services was around one-third by 1980 (Günal 2008). Although the Law on Socialization of Health Services in 1961 attempted to establish a universal, citizenship-based, social insurance system for all health care services, this plan never came to fruition. Instead, universal access remained limited to basic services such as vaccination and prenatal and antenatal care.

The developmentalist era in Turkey also witnessed sweeping demographic and cultural transformations. The political alignments of the Cold War initiated a set of social, political, and economic changes that rendered the early Turkish state's isolationist approach toward the countryside obsolete. Turkey became a strong ally of the US in polarized global politics by joining NATO in 1952 and hosting American military bases on its soil. In return, the US granted Turkey, along with other European countries, Marshall Funds to facilitate Turkey's incorporation into the global economy, encourage economic growth, and thwart the further spread of communism. Accordingly, the proponents of the modernization theory, a pivotal intellectual weapon of the US empire, categorized Turkey as "un(der)developed" (Adalet 2018). Academics and state officials proposed a series of strategies, including investments in highways and agricultural machinery, thereby helping the country generate wealth and prosperity without straying off into alternative paths to capitalist order such as communism and socialism.

The most immediate outcome of the agricultural mechanization was the decreasing need for male labor in rural areas, a development that coincided with the growing demand for labor in the industry and service sectors of large cities (Özbay 1995). These parallel developments ignited an unprecedented rural-to-urban migration, elevating the share of the urban population from 25 percent in 1950 to 43.9 percent in 1980 and 59 percent in 1990 (Yilmaz 2015). Migrants from the same villages clustered in the same neighborhoods

in cities; built gecekondu (makeshift houses) on public land; established communities according to their lifestyles, ethnic identities, and cultural values; and
developed their separate clientelist networks (hemşehrilik) (Erder 1999). These
networks, at least in the early decades, provided new urban dwellers lacking education, skills, or economic capital with an opportunity for social mobility and
a sense of belonging to both the villages they left behind and their new homes.

As for social security for the migrants, due to the difficulty of securing
employment in the formal manufacturing sector, many remained outside the
formal social insurance system. The migrant neighborhoods initially lacked
basic infrastructure and social services such as roads, sanitation, and schools
as well as health services. As the beginning of the multiparty system in 1950
opened the possibility for an "informal pact" between political parties and the
gecekondu dwellers, the migrants began to acquire services from municipalities
by deploying their electoral status as leverage: they voted collectively for parties
promising to meet their basic needs (Bugra 2007). The migrants' pragmatic use
of elections contributed to their ongoing stigmatization in the eyes of original
urban residents. These residents regarded migrants' leverage in elections as a
sign of corruption and lack of autonomy, stigmatizing the migrants as less
than full citizens.[2]

Given the limited welfare coverage of the 1960s, philanthropic associations and benevolent individuals unsurprisingly continued to be at the
forefront of managing poverty, including providing mass circumcisions for
low-income families in Turkey. Starting in the 1960s, mass circumcisions
in cities began to be organized and funded by civil society organizations or
sometimes municipalities (though, as I discuss in chapter 5, municipalities'
involvement in male circumcision became widespread only with the rise of
pro-Islamist parties in the 1990s). As in the case of imperial circumcisions
in the Ottoman era, the organizers provided gifts and circumcision outfits
for children and met the expenses for the operations. Health officers and, to
a decreasing degree, itinerant circumcisers tapped themselves into these mass
circumcisions, which went hand in hand with the consolidation of calculative
reasoning and the monetization of male circumcision.

MONETIZATION AND CALCULATION

I talked to Sünnetçi Çetin, a sixty-two-year-old health officer, at his clinic
in a city in Central Anatolia. He had been circumcising boys for forty years
and worked in two different cities before he settled in the current one. I was
waiting for the interview outside of his office as he was providing information
to parents about their son's circumcision. After having overheard them talking

about the payment method, I looked around for a price signboard for circumcision in the clinic but could not see one. During my research, I came across only one clinic that put out such a board for public view.

After the parents left, he and I sat down for the interview. Fifteen to twenty minutes into the interview, Sünnetçi Çetin, unprompted by me, highlighted his charity activities:

ÇETİN: I circumcise cops' sons for free here. I also circumcise orphans for free every year.
AUTHOR: How much do you normally charge for one kid?
ÇETİN: Let's not talk about that.

And as we continued our conversation, I wanted to ask about the difficulties of performing circumcision:

AUTHOR: Was there any aspect of this job you don't like?
ÇETİN: It is not always economically satisfying. Families spend all the money on the celebration, food, alcohol, etc., but when it comes to the operation, they start bargaining with you.
AUTHOR: So, you have a set price for each circumcision, but are also open to negotiation?
ÇETİN: Yes, sometimes. It depends on how business is going. Private hospitals are charging families more. Think about it. What is the difference between my circumcision and their circumcision? Nothing.
AUTHOR: Was the situation the same at the first two places you worked?
ÇETİN: No, because there are more circumcisers here and you must keep the price lower.
AUTHOR: I guess families also have more bargaining power, right?
ÇETİN: Yes.

While Sünnetçi Çetin circumcised police officers' sons free of charge in gratitude for their services, an annual tradition that some health officers followed, his other charity activities were meant to meet low-income families' needs. Both types of events drew media attention, providing an opportunity for him to craft an altruistic image—an image that accounted as much for his eagerness to talk about these events as his refusal to answer my question about the prices of his circumcision services.

However, Sünnetçi Çetin was also resentful of middle-class families for bargaining over prices, a routine that signaled, in his view, an ill-informed approach to male circumcision: by trying to lower the price, these families, he thought, underappreciated the significance of the operation to boys' health. Some of my other interviewees also shared Sünnetçi Çetin's sentiments about bargaining, as it contradicted a core moral component of their habitus: the disavowal of economic motives ("We are not in this for money").

Bargaining became more common when health officers began to medicalize the practice in the 1960s and started setting the price for circumcision in advance. This was a new payment method, as until then families had been compensating itinerant circumcisers in a nonstandardized manner. Chapter 1 showed that when an itinerant circumciser walked into a village, families brought their sons to him without an appointment. Itinerant circumcisers did not establish a fixed price for circumcision either: payments tended to be irregular, unpredictable, informal, and collective. One payment method commonly used by itinerant circumcisers was to circulate a tray:

AUTHOR: When you went to villages, how were you compensated?
SERHAT: The villagers were adorning a tea tray and circulating it around. Men who were part of the community and were invited to circumcisions were all chipping in. How much is a pack of cigarettes, now? Say, ten thousand Turkish liras. If everyone gave you a pack of cigarettes' worth of money, that would be a lot. Sometimes I collected a lot. Other times, it was not much. But we were fourteen siblings, and the money my father made from circumcision was enough for all of us.

Serhat, a son of an itinerant circumciser, went to villages with his father, though he himself never performed circumcision. He and his father did not know how much they would collect from a village in total, as they had no control over how much boys' families, let alone other villagers, would put on the tray. Due to their strong ties with locals, they trusted that locals would give them enough to be able to make a living as a large family.

Itinerant circumcisers' economic reasoning was, in other words, not rationalized, as they did not seek to transform male circumcision into a calculable and predictable business activity. My interviewees said that they did not know how many boys they would circumcise or how much they would be able to collect from each village. Nor did they make any attempt to set a price for a circumcision. Hence, no room for bargaining. Compensation in nonmonetary terms such as food, chicken, or clothes was not uncommon between families and itinerant circumcisers. These circumcisers typically showed no interest in expanding into new territories or scaling up their circumcision activities either.

However, most of my interviewees, including itinerant circumcisers, later adopted a more stringent calculative reasoning and approach. I talked to Sünnetçi Şafak in a town in northern Turkey that in recent decades has experienced a large-scale expansion of both rural-to-urban migration and immigration to foreign countries. Sünnetçi Şafak did not have a license and learned to use medical methods (both local anesthesia and sutures) from a health officer with whom he collaborated for a short time. When I asked him about his compensation method, he responded:

ŞAFAK: In the past, a circumciser used to hold a tray with a towel [a gift from a boy's family] on the top of it, and then villagers circulated the tray among themselves. Everyone was chipping in however much they could or wanted. Then, the circumciser would begin to perform the circumcision.

AUTHOR: Is this how you used to get paid, too?

ŞAFAK: At first, I did. They sometimes gave me only chicken or a T-shirt. But then I fixed the price for each circumcision.

AUTHOR: Why did you do that?

ŞAFAK: The number of boys declined because of migration, and I wanted to make money. So, I fixed the price per child.

AUTHOR: And you started settling on the price in advance?

ŞAFAK: Yes.

AUTHOR: Was there no bargaining?

ŞAFAK: Sometimes there was. Especially if the family had more than one boy who needed to be circumcised. I was asking less for the second boy. I also started working only by appointment.

AUTHOR: Why?

ŞAFAK: Well, there were expenses such as gas, anesthesia, suture, etc., that I had to think about. This is not like old circumcision. I have to buy supplies and drive to circumcisions myself. I don't go to circumcisions on foot.

The decreasing demands for male circumcision due to (im)migration, the costs of the new medical techniques, and the desire to make money all urged Sünnetçi Şafak to make his transactions with families more predictable, standard, and calculable. He could no longer afford the vagaries of the traditional method if he wished to sustain his now medicalized practice. Unlike Sünnetçi Şafak, who set the price for his services himself, some circumcisers allowed the families to decide on the price insofar as the proposed price surpassed the costs. In doing so, they wanted to create an intimacy with families, signaling to them that money was not their primary concern. Money signified both a potentially corrupting force and a medium for "connected lives" (Zelizer 2005).

Another factor that pushed for a more rational method of delivering circumcision services was the intensified competition between itinerant circumcisers and health officers. I talked to Barber Ekrem at his barbershop in an eastern city of Turkey, where he began to work as an apprentice for a barber at the age of ten and learned to perform circumcision from his master. His master watched the first circumcision that Ekrem performed, which was at the age of twenty-two, and approved his competence. When I asked Sünnetçi Ekrem about his compensation method, he said:

EKREM: There was this custom of holding a tray . . . the largest amount was given by the immediate family: father, mother, uncle, and the rest would give an amount suitable to their budget. That was the custom. Then, health officers showed up; some of them opened clinics, and families were asking, "I have two children, how much would I pay for circumcision?" Health officers were cutting off for a set price, and then we also began to do the same. With the old system, we were sometimes having more and sometimes less money on the tray. We did not know how much we would make. But we were still going, saying, "It is nasip [destiny or luck]." Then, of course, it became fixed.

AUTHOR: Did health officers give you a hard time?

EKREM: Yes, because we did not have a license. Of course, it was all for the sake of profit.

AUTHOR: How much were you charging?

EKREM: It depends. Look at all these circumcisions [he shows me his notebook for bookkeeping]. It says "bedava" [for free]. I performed many circumcisions free of charge [he covers the prices for other circumcisions with his other hand].

The increasing competition from health officers combined with medicalization pressured Sünnetçi Ekrem to treat circumcisions on an individual basis. The basic reference point of his circumcision activity shifted from *village* to *family* as he embraced the fee-for-service model. In the old model, the provision of circumcision supplies (for instance, herbs) was barely monetized. With medicalization, he now had to buy sutures and anesthesia and sterilize his instruments regularly. He fixed the price for each circumcision, which also created room for bargaining.

The developmentalist era in male circumcision was characterized by both material and ideational changes about the practice: health officers, followed by itinerant circumcisers, infused the practice with a calculative logic, thereby transforming it into a biomedical commodity. All these changes, as hinted at by Sünnetçi Ekrem, who did not want to disclose the prices of his circumcisions, ran the risk of coming into conflict with an important aspect of professional habitus: an altruistic self- and public image based on the normative orientation to serving others. In that regard, performing mass circumcision became a crucial way to avoid this risk.

MASS CIRCUMCISION

From the 1960s onwards, mass circumcisions were typically funded in cities and towns by charitable organizations, private companies, associations, trade unions, newspapers, children protection agencies, and sometimes the Turkish army and municipalities. For operations, hundreds of boys dressed in circumcision outfits were gathered in outdoor settings (for instance, schoolyards and parks) or large indoor venues (for instance, sporting facilities). Circumcisers performed these circumcisions, either with the help of assistants or on their own. Sometimes two or three circumcisers worked together and, when they had not agreed to perform the operations for free, split the fees. To get the lowest price per circumcision, sponsors occasionally shopped around and asked circumcisers about their fees in advance, though many circumcisers mentioned to me that they charged sponsors only enough to cover operation costs.

Mass circumcisions of the developmentalist era provided circumcisers like Sünnetçi Metin with visibility and reputation among locals and even sometimes coverage in local newspapers. I contacted Sünnetçi Metin in a city in northwestern Turkey through another health officer, Sünnetçi İnanç from the same region. İnanç suggested that I should go to the pharmacy run by Sünnetçi Metin's children to learn his whereabouts. When I arrived at the pharmacy, his daughter sent me to the coffeehouse where Sünnetçi Metin usually hung out, played card games, and socialized with others. The pharmacy was in a six-story building, and later in our interview, Sünnetçi Metin mentioned that he owned the entire building and had purchased it with his additional income from male circumcision.

I went straight from the pharmacy to the coffeehouse and met Sünnetçi Metin, an eighty-three-year-old health officer. After he ordered us tea, he and I sat down for the interview. As I was explaining to him my research, he interrupted me:

METİN: Did İnanç tell you that I won first place in 1970?
AUTHOR: First place in what?
METİN: Did he tell you that?
AUTHOR: No.
METİN: That's why they call me "Jet Sünnetçi" (Jet Circumciser). In 1970, I circumcised 120 kids within three hours. I had assistants, but I cut all of them off on my own. İnanç was there, too.

AUTHOR: Oh! I did not know they called you "Jet Sünnetçi." Who organized this event?

METIN: The Child Protection Agency. Then, I appeared in newspapers as "Jet Sünnetçi."

Jet Sünnetçi Metin graduated from a Village Institute (see chapter 2) and began to perform circumcision in 1951. He and Sünnetçi İnanç performed some of the mass circumcisions together. Sünnetçi İnanç had been circumcising boys since 1966 without, unlike Sünnetçi Metin, formal medical education. He instead received a license from a state hospital after he had assisted Sünnetçi Metin for seventeen years. I interviewed İnanç before Metin, and İnanç had also mentioned the same mass circumcision, leaving out the "jet sünnetçi" part:

İNANÇ: You do not even have time to eat. We were just putting some powder on penises and then letting boys go. We did not have enough time to dress the incisions. It was like a bus terminal. Children were lined up and were being held tight by elderly people. We were cutting one [foreskin] off and moving to another one. Once Metin and I circumcised 120 children inside a park.

AUTHOR: Was that event the one organized by the municipality? I think I read about it.

İNANÇ: No, by the Child Protection Agency. Children of poor families [fakir fukara çocukları]. 120 children. It was one child per minute. It was like a factory. We were doing our best to be careful, but it was nothing like the circumcisions today. But ask anyone here, they would know me. Go ahead, ask anyone [he points toward people around us]. They would know me, because I circumcised many poor kids for free. If the kids are orphans, I don't charge anything. If the family is on minimum wage, I do it for free. How could they then pay for rent if they also paid for circumcision? If I cared about money, people would not like or respect me the way they do now. Once, a very good friend of mine wanted to have their sons circumcised in a nearby town. I asked him if he knew any poor families in that area. I also circumcised their boys. Ten kids. Their parents were crying and thanking me. If I were concerned about profit, I would not do it for free.

For Sünnetçi İnanç and Sünnetçi Metin, performing mass circumcision free of charge was a way to establish a social network and follow a moral code: helping the poor. By performing these circumcisions, they could express gratitude for the acceptance they received from locals and strengthen their sense of belonging as sünnetçi within the community. Both circumcisers thought that a circumciser with a profit-seeking attitude would be rejected by locals—a concern clearly articulated by Sünnetçi İnanç when he said, "If I cared about money, people would not like or respect me the way they do now." Yet, they also wanted to earn money from the practice. Mass circumcisions served as a platform to manage this tension, as these charity events allowed them to accumulate social capital, disavow their economic motives, and maintain an altruistic self- and public image.

Performing mass circumcision granted health officers an advantage over itinerant circumcisers, as well. Sünnetçi Odhan, a sixty-three-year-old health officer, had performed mass circumcision for decades and had quit it a few years before the interview. He brought up mass circumcisions when we were talking about a confrontation he once had with barbers and some locals:

ODHAN: Barbers did not numb it. I was using local anesthesia. People then started coming to me for circumcision. Would they ever hold a barber on a par with me? No.

AUTHOR: So, families accepted your method right away?

ODHAN: Well, not all of them. Some people were ignorant, uneducated. There was also almost no mass media. There wasn't even a radio. Kids now have all the opportunities. Oh, and I circumcised thousands of poor boys for free in the initial years of doing this job. I performed most of the mass operations free of charge.

AUTHOR: Did performing mass circumcisions make people lean towards you rather than barbers?

ODHAN: Not really . . . well, sort of. I became known here. You perform circumcisions, and other people see it. They see you at celebrations. They see how boys recover from circumcisions and get up and dance. There were ministers, health ministers, who attended these events. Once a health minister gathered everyone, including the governor, brought them to me, and said, "Look, this is our circumciser. He performs the best procedures." Then, photos were taken. But I got no money from that event. Their blessing was good enough for me.

AUTHOR: Who was organizing these events?

ODHAN: Until the beginning of the 1980s, workers. It was labor unions here. We circumcised their kids too. Once, it was two of us, and the other health officer came to me, complaining that he had no one to circumcise. And I looked back—there was a long line of boys behind me. They preferred me. They all were waiting to be circumcised by me. People knew me. But I said to the other health officer, "I can't do all of them. We have to share them." I also circumcised poor boys outside of mass circumcisions. I was going to villages to circumcise kids. There were also poor families. They had nothing, neither money nor land.

They were asking, "I also have two boys. Can you circumcise them?" I was circumcising them, too. It was for charity. I know what poverty is like. I grew up poor. How can I not understand them? I remember having gone to bed hungry on many nights. Why would I not circumcise them? I treated everyone well.

Sünnetçi Odhan's self-portrayal as a popular circumciser suggests that performing mass circumcisions for free was an important route toward gaining status and a competitive advantage over other circumcisers. Like all health officers, Sünnetçi Odhan came from a poor family and had transformed this biographical fact into a powerful affective fiction imbuing his performances of mass circumcision—an otherwise mundane procedure—with an intimate feeling of unity with the poor ("How can I not understand them?). This powerful fiction, commonly used by many health officers, reinforced the givenness of their motives for performing mass circumcision: "Why would I not circumcise them?" By not charging for mass circumcisions, Sünnetçi Odhan posited sentimentality against money and the calculative logic that money represented. After all, families' "blessing" was good enough for him.

The symbolic significance of the imperial circumcisions, as mentioned earlier, was characterized by a disavowal of political interest. Imperial circumcisions helped foster an imagined unity between the sultan and subjects, leading the latter to feel invested in, taken care of, and represented in the larger polity. In the 1960s, health officers' goal to drive itinerant circumcisers from the field inevitably raised the question of pursuing economic self-interest, which conflicted with the altruistic image that these practitioners aimed to project. Accordingly, by performing mass male circumcisions, health officers assumed a share of the original sovereign benevolence, now based on the disavowal of not political but economic interests, thereby improving or maintaining their footing in communities.

Besides social and symbolic capital, mass circumcisions helped health officers accumulate another form of capital: cultural capital. As demonstrated in chapter 2, young health officers who finished their medical education with little to no experience in circumcision faced competition from much more experienced circumcisers (itinerant circumcisers and senior health officers). To address this problem, they made short-term arrangements with senior circumcisers, including itinerant circumcisers, who helped them acquire experience as well as connections with locals. Similarly, mass circumcisions presented a very efficient training opportunity for these health officers to improve their skills, as they could circumcise hundreds of boys within a short period. Health officer Hakan, who co-owned a clinic with his father in Istanbul, first watched his father, who was also a licensed circumciser. I asked him about his training:

HAKAN: When I was twelve or thirteen years old, my father said, "Come on, no need to be lazy and waste your time. You are coming to [do] circumcisions with me." He was circumcising boys, and I was watching and assisting him, giving him tools, etc. Circumcision was a good job. People were showing him respect, and he was making good money. He was in high demand around here. He was working very hard. I studied medicine for two years at a university and then started performing circumcisions too. I especially improved my skills at these [mass] circumcisions. I performed them for five years.

AUTHOR: Where were the mass circumcisions taking place?

HAKAN: They were outdoors. The organizers were setting up tents. My father once even performed them in a stadium. But of course, you must be very fast, like seventy boys within an hour and a half—think about it . . . it was that fast. You inevitably develop your skills very quickly.

The crowded nature of mass circumcisions appealed to young Hakan, who wanted to take over his father's business as soon as possible. Improving circumcision skills, especially cutting skills, takes practice, and mass circumcisions helped him significantly shorten the training period. After his father's sudden death, Sünnetçi Hakan became one of the well-known circumcisers in the area.

Another aspect of mass circumcisions during the developmentalist era was the lack of surveillance over circumcisers. Contrary to middle-class families, low-income families did not have control over how and by whom their sons were circumcised, as these decisions were left to the discretion of sponsors and health officers. And sponsors sometimes recruited young health officers to lower the costs for these circumcisions, as those health officers were eager to improve their skills, albeit not ready to perform circumcision independently. Sünnetçi Kerim, a senior health officer, was rather disturbed by the fact that some of his assistants who were not, in Kerim's view, qualified yet to perform circumcision on their own used mass circumcisions as an opportunity to expedite their training. His account portrays a striking class-based contrast between individual circumcisions and mass circumcisions:

KERİM: Now, I am a circumciser, and I will circumcise a child. You want to learn how to perform circumcisions. How are you going to learn? I can't let you circumcise these [nonpoor] children, because his parents trust me. It would be inappropriate for me to let you circumcise him. Mass circumcisions are different. Hundreds of children were circumcised, and there was sometimes more than one circumciser present. It was so chaotic that no one knew what the others were doing [kim kime dum duma]. No one can tell who the circumciser is and who the assistant is. He [his assistant] could take advantage of the situation, circumcise these children, and gain experience in a short time. That's why some of my assistants performed these operations for free.

AUTHOR: What do you mean? Can you elaborate on this?

KERİM: Imagine that you are rich and want to organize a mass circumcision event for five hundred children. Whom would you hire for this job? You would ask who would do it for free, right? Who would perform those circumcisions for free? Of course, someone who wants to improve his cutting skills. Many people accepted to perform these circumcisions for this reason in the past. Many mistakes were made, and many children suffered. Maybe those children still suffer.

Sünnetçi Kerim, unlike many of my interviewees, did not want to perform mass circumcisions free of charge, and in such cases sponsors might choose instead to work with a circumciser who would. Sünnetçi Kerim believed that the lack of regulation over circumcisers at mass circumcisions caused unnecessary suffering in boys. Unlike at circumcisions for the nonpoor, circumcisers at mass circumcisions did not interact with individual families but rather only with sponsors, and thus would not be held responsible by families for the mistakes they might make during procedures.

Like Sünnetçi Kerim, Sünnetçi Mustafa had also felt frustrated over the organization of mass circumcisions. Sünnetçi Mustafa, a senior health officer, performed only those mass circumcisions sponsored by religiously motivated humanitarian associations outside of Turkey. These associations brought circumcisers to foreign Muslim countries, where they organized circumcision events including the operations for low-income families. When I asked Sünnetçi Mustafa why he did not perform mass circumcision in Turkey, he said:

I did a couple of them, but then I didn't want to. I don't think mass circumcisions are safe in Turkey. Those who want to organize mass circumcisions here prefer whoever would do it for free. They stopped coming to me. Why? Because when they did, I said I wanted money, this much money per child. Then to whom would they go? Who would do it for free? They are many people who are eager to learn it. There was a lot of trouble because of that.

Gender, class, and race often, as medical sociologists and historians show, determine who becomes vulnerable to ethically problematic medical research, training, and clinical trials, sowing the seeds of distrust in modern science and medicine within some segments of the society—for instance, women, the poor, and black people (Benjamin 2013; Cahill 2001; Gamble 1993; Humphrey

1973; Petryna 2009). Similarly, the lack of financial means to afford individual circumcisions stripped the low-income families of any control over how their sons' circumcisions were to be performed, making them vulnerable to the consequences of health officers' shortcuts for improving their circumcision skills. Health officers' accumulation of cultural capital (circumcision skills), in other words, came at the cost of quality medical care for low-income families.

Overall, three motivations behind circumcisers' involvement in mass circumcisions could be observed during the developmentalist era. The main reason was the symbolic significance of mass circumcisions, as these charity events enabled circumcisers (particularly, health officers) to disavow their motives for economic profits, foster an altruistic self- and public image as the carer of the poor in medical terms, and accrue public visibility, prestige, and recognition. Thus, health officers during this era transformed themselves into not only Fenni Sünnetçi but also the Benevolent Circumciser who carried a share of the sovereign benevolence once embodied and monopolized by the sultans in the Ottoman era.

The second reason for health officers to participate in mass circumcision events was to gain cultural capital. The sponsoring organizations helped health officers further cope with the mismatch between their level of skills and their desire for increasing their power in the field. Mass circumcision events stood in contrast to circumcisions for the nonpoor, where boys received individualized attention from circumcisers. The events instead rendered poor bodies anonymous: it was, as circumcisers mentioned, hard for them to distinguish one child from another.

The same anonymity emerging from gathering boys in the same location also made these operations a potential source of economic capital for health officers, though most circumcisers performed them either at no charge or at cost. The economic appeal of mass circumcisions had to do with the fact that health officers could circumcise more boys within a much shorter time than they would otherwise. While regular individual circumcisions for the nonpoor could take from ten to fifteen minutes, circumcisers allocated only two or three minutes, or sometimes even less, for each child at these mass events. Although they lowered their fixed price per circumcision for mass circumcisions, the size of these events made the event financially worthwhile for them.[3]

The medicalization of the 1960s led to the inculcation of a rational and calculative disposition toward male circumcision, and circumcisers identified themselves with the new normative understanding of Sünnetçi only by marking a distance from it through mass circumcisions. Not doing so could harm their status within communities. They thus downplayed economic interests and idealized benevolence. However, the image of the Benevolent Circumciser during the developmentalist era was not immune to contradictions either.

"MASS MASSACRES"

Mass circumcisions also generated new contradictions concerning medical care, as practitioners often felt that they were violating the moral principle of "do not harm" by performing these operations. Sünnetçi Emin, a health officer, talked about the mass circumcisions he had performed in the past with a regretful tone in his voice:

EMIN: For normal operations, I was applying two or three stitches, and the incision was healing much faster. I was also performing mass circumcisions. I remember once I circumcised 156 children in two hours on my own. They were placed on the floor, lying next to each other. I smoked only one cigarette during that time.

AUTHOR: Did you use local anesthesia and sutures for those circumcisions as well?

EMIN: No, I just used a coolant. For local anesthesia, I would need another three or five minutes. I was circumcising each boy in a minute or so. Then I stopped performing mass circumcisions.

AUTHOR: Why?

EMIN: It was too risky for us and the kids. The conditions were not good.

As chapter 2 discussed, local anesthesia and sutures lengthened the necessary amount of time a circumciser needed for what he considered a safe operation: namely, painless circumcision without postoperative complications. Due to limited time during mass circumcisions, Sünnetçi Emin could not meet what were then the standards for biomedical care and fulfill his moral obligation for the boys. He also expressed concerns regarding the risk of mass circumcisions for his own health—a well-grounded concern, given that it was not, as multiple health officers mentioned, uncommon to have accidents (for instance, cuts on hands) during the operations. Sünnetçi Emin, especially, highlighted the risk of exposure to blood-borne diseases such as Hepatitis C.

Many other health officers also decided at some point not to perform mass circumcisions, for the same reasons mentioned by Sünnetçi Emin. Sünnetçi Mahmut, a fifty-five-year-old health officer, was one of the few health officers who had also received a college degree. His nephew was the first person he circumcised: "Of course, I was nervous, because we had seen circumcision theoretically at school, but not much practically," he said. After gaining confidence by performing individual circumcisions, he began to perform mass circumcisions as well, but later he stopped participating in these events:

> There was no sterilization, and as health professionals, we place a high premium on hygiene. Why? Because we think that sterilization is an effective protection against infections. But you can't really think about hygiene at mass circumcisions. You have a couple of instruments and you must clean them with solutions as you go, instead of using new instruments for each operation. So, I did not want to do it. After I quit, I agreed to perform these operations a couple of more times, only if there were twenty or thirty kids to circumcise. But then I stopped doing it altogether.

Medical disinfection, as shown in the previous chapters, was a routine practice that health officers introduced to male circumcision and was also adopted by some itinerant circumcisers. Given that traditional circumcisions were seen as lacking any concern regarding sterilization, this method of protection from infections and diseases contributed to health officers' efforts in representing themselves as the only legitimate practitioners. Failing to bring the mass operations up to the normative hygiene standards of the time, as in the case of Sünnetçi Mahmut, could thus take an emotional toll on health officers.

Besides routine disinfection, follow-ups were another important stage of medicalized male circumcisions. Many health officers mentioned sleepless nights after performing operations at the beginning of their careers, worrying about postoperative complications. While this worry subsided over time, if not completely disappearing, follow-ups became a permanent component of health officers' circumcisions. The importance of this care explains why the lack of regular follow-ups also alienated some health officers from mass circumcisions.

Sünnetçi Nedim was one of the health officers who, once graduated from medical school, watched both itinerant circumcisers and senior health officers to improve his skills. He was first assigned to a Kurdish city and then requested reassignment to a western city to be geographically close to his wife's family. He performed individual and mass circumcisions in both cities:

NEDİM: I went to mass circumcisions in both cities. Then, I thought about these circumcisions [silence]. I am a medical professional, and the rate of transmission of many diseases, especially Hepatitis B, syphilis, and similar ones, was very high at these operations. You also don't do your regular follow-ups. You do not see them again. One day, I decided not to do it. I promised myself that I would not go to mass circumcisions. They are still calling me about it. I say no. I call them [mass circumcisions] *mass massacre.*

AUTHOR: Oh, really?

NEDİM: Yeah, because there is no sterilization, disinfection there. When I go to [individual] circumcisions, I prepare tool kits for each kid and have a sterilizer. I would not go to any circumcision without placing my instruments in the sterilizer. You couldn't do that at mass circumcisions.

"Mass massacre" (Toplu Katliam) is an emotionally charged phrase that my other interviewees also used to condemn mass circumcisions. It conveys anger, frustration, and guilt over the potential harm done to boys. The phrase appeared widely in mass media around the 1990s, drawing an analogy between mass circumcisions and the religious practice of sacrificing animals on Eid al-Adha. The annual sacrifice of an animal (for instance, sheep) in Islam represents acts of both devotion to Allah and a sharing of wealth as owners distribute the slaughtered animals between their family, neighbors, and the needy members of the community. The ritual in Turkey typically takes place in outdoor settings and involves reading a verse from the Quran, pinning down an animal and slitting its throat, and draining the blood into a hole on the ground. The blood also gets smeared on the foreheads of the owner's family.

Over the last three decades, the ritual has become a matter of public disputes among religious leaders and scholars, health authorities, politicians enthusiastic about the country's prospect of joining the EU, and animal rights activists. These actors have raised concerns regarding the unnecessary suffering caused in animals by inexperienced butchers and improper venues (for instance, bathrooms in homes or streets rather than government-provided facilities) where animals have often been slaughtered in large and crowded cities. The mismanagement of the ritual could not only, it was claimed, cause public health problems but also create images of violence and aggression that had no place in Islam. Others proposed that the ritual be replaced with forms of charity that did not involve animals, such as providing a scholarship for students in need. At the same time, newspapers published photos of pools of blood on the street or in the sea, presented as distasteful scenes caused by irresponsible families, sellers, and butchers. These concerned actors fought to change the aesthetics and ethics of the ritual, making it compatible with what they deemed modern, safe, and humane standards.

With the phrase "mass massacre," health officers compared mass circumcisions to the annual Muslim Feast of Sacrifice, alluding to all the problems that the critiques of the feast pointed out. Health officers, often angrily, said, "These are children, not sheep!" or "Kids were like sacrificial sheep"—remarks intended to dramatize the care-related problems observed at mass circumcisions. Behind the moral overtone of the phrase "mass massacre" lies the perceived mistreatment of animals during the feast: just as animals were passive helpless victims of abuse, so were poor boys who were circumcised too fast under unsanitary conditions.

While all the senior health officers I interviewed raised concerns and expressed bitter feelings about mass circumcisions, some continued to perform mass operations in a new way: they introduced an appointment system—the same system that was already in effect for individual circumcisions. Sünnetçi Selim began to perform circumcision in 1972 and was assigned to two other places before he permanently settled in his current city in western Turkey. He performed individual and mass circumcisions alike in all these three places, which were located in three different regions. He learned to perform circumcision from another senior health officer, with whom he went to mass circumcisions as well. In our conversation, he prided himself on how he had adapted his mentor's method of performing the operations:

SELİM: I carried his tool bag for two years. He did not want to teach me first. This is a very risky job. If you break a leg of a table, you can replace it. But if you make a mistake circumcising a kid, there is no fixing for it. That's why he did not want me to do it, and I understood him. But then I circumcised my nephew, and that's how I started it.

AUTHOR: What about mass circumcisions? Did you ever do it?

SELİM: I did, but not anymore. To be honest, I am not in favor of it. You use the same instrument again and again without sterilizing it. There is not enough hygiene. It is not like a normal circumcision. Later, I started doing it differently, though others also followed me.

AUTHOR: How?

SELİM: For instance, once the municipality organized a mass circumcision event. I wanted to perform them at home. They said I should circumcise only one or two kids in public as part of celebrations. I did that. Then I got their addresses and went to their homes. I finished all of them within two days.

AUTHOR: Where were you performing these circumcisions before?

SELİM: Outdoor venues. They sometimes set up tents. But all of the places were too chaotic.

Health officers possessed what low-income families lacked: decision-making power over the methods and organization of mass circumcisions. As a respected member of the community, Sünnetçi Selim used his prestige to change the long-standing tradition of mass circumcisions in his area to make it compatible with what he considered safe male circumcision. He individualized mass operations, while the anonymous nature of the celebrations where families, local politicians, sponsors, and local media gathered remained the same.

Like Sünnetçi Selim, Sünnetçi Fahri also mentioned a change in the organization of mass circumcision over the years:

FAHRİ: We changed how we did mass circumcisions at some point. It is nothing like you used to see on TV. In the past, these circumcisions were done in outdoor settings, like cafes. I understand, because they [the sponsors] wanted it to be as cheap as possible. But there was always a big crowd and chaos. We said we would agree to prepare a list of boys who needed to be circumcised and get their families' addresses and phone numbers (in case we could not find the addresses). Then, we call them. We call them and give them specific dates so that they know when we are coming. It is still called "mass circumcisions," but we instead go to their places. Oh, please don't get me wrong. We are not seeking any benefits in doing this.

AUTHOR: What do you mean?

FAHRİ: You know, in case you would think that, since we go to their homes, we would ask for money. We would never do that. We are doing this for charity. They [the sponsors] only cover our expenses. This is meant to be our contribution, our support for these people. Instead of being with strangers, kids get circumcised in their family environment. I think this is better and more successful. In doing so, we hope that this will be a pleasant memory for them. They would say: "They came to our houses and circumcised our children." They were grateful for that.

In his self-presentation as a medical actor, Sünnetçi Fahri was worried about giving away the impression of having an ulterior economic motive lurking behind his mass circumcision activities. He framed his mass circumcision activities as a contribution to the community wherein he forged his sense of belonging as a circumciser, and he highlighted the superiority of the appointment system over the old model in ensuring efficiency, safety, and social cohesion. With the new system, he and Sünnetçi Selim could spread out the vast number of operations over a few days and perform them without a rush. Moreover, low-income families could now have their sons circumcised in their homes with relatives and neighbors. The appointment system provided, as in the case of individual circumcisions for the nonpoor, an intimate space for these families to celebrate what they regarded as a milestone in their sons' lives without mingling with strangers.

Instead of, or in addition to, families' homes, other circumcisers sometimes scheduled appointments for circumcisions to take place at their clinics.

I interviewed Sünnetçi Bahri, a health officer, at his clinic, and as we were talking about the health risks involved in male circumcision in general, he brought up mass circumcisions:

BAHRİ: The kid's sexual life is in your hands. His self-confidence. Not everyone should do this job. We are thus against mass circumcisions. We even made comments on this issue in newspapers.

AUTHOR: I was going to ask that. Have you ever done it?

BAHRİ: I did and still do it, but not outdoors anymore. They either come here or I go to each boy's home. For example, suppose I get a hundred kids. I don't do it all at once at the same place. The celebration happens at the same place later. In the past, we were doing it on the grass, parks, gyms, wedding halls on the floor. We stopped doing that. Now it is different. We can't even call it "mass circumcisions" anymore. We can call it "mass celebration," but not "circumcision."

AUTHOR: Because boys are not circumcised at the same place?

BAHRİ: No, they can be circumcised at the same place, but not at the same time. I have a hundred kids. Five of them come today and the other five kids come tomorrow. Ten kids come the next day. And they all come here.

By dividing mass circumcisions into separate time slots, Sünnetçi Bahri sought to transform, with the support of the sponsors, "mass massacres" into "mass celebrations," targeting the morally disturbing aspects of an approach to circumcisions that delivered less-than-ideal biomedical care. The introduction of an appointment-based model into mass circumcisions was, therefore, an outcome of his critical and moral reflection on these operations, which he had also come to see as chaotic and harmful to the health of boys and circumcisers alike.

Unlike their colleagues who shared the same nagging feeling of regret but responded to it by quitting performing mass operations, Sünnetçi Bahri and some of the other health officers instead improvised a new method of delivery—inspired by individual circumcision services—to address class-based inequalities while continuing to accumulate the associated symbolic profits. Health officers' distinct responses to the same troubling situation suggest that the symbolic profits associated with mass circumcisions did not inherently coincide with a particular organizational model, even though each model rested on the same distinction between the poor and the nonpoor.

DISAVOWAL

As economic sociologists argue, calculative logic and the economic notions of rationality and self-interest associated with capitalism are not intrinsic to human nature; rather, they are historical constructions (Bourdieu 2005; Polanyi 2001; Weber 1946). As such, these dispositions are cultivated and often must gain legitimacy in the eyes of the public. Starting in the 1960s, health officers began to commodify medical male circumcision and made economic self-interest, calculation, and predictability the dominant characteristics of the field. From their perspective, the old methods of compensation, where the price for circumcision was not fixed, were erratic and arbitrary. In contrast, the fee-for-service model could lessen such uncertainties and thus was more conducive to accumulating profits.

Yet, an overt profit-seeking disposition would also be disliked by communities. Therefore, at the same time, health officers became increasingly involved in mass circumcision events organized for low-income families and typically circumcised boys free of charge at these events to establish strong ties with communities. In doing so, they invoked what economic sociologist Viviana Zelizer (2011) calls "hostile worlds": money, instrumental rationality, and commodification on the one hand, and sentimentality and intimacy on the other hand. Although Zelizer mainly coined this phrase to disclose a false dichotomy observed in scholarly writings about the market, a dichotomy that suggests that the market inevitably corrupts sentimentality, she also acknowledged that people (like health officers, in our case), via discourses and practices, regularly invoke these hostile worlds to make connections with others.

Pierre Bourdieu's notion of "disavowal," if understood in psychoanalytical terms,[4] can, I suggest, capture the pressure generally associated with the ambivalence of the economic subjectivity of the 1960s as exemplified in male circumcision in Turkey. From a Bourdieusian framework, mass circumcisions could be seen as a form of symbolic capital based on the "disavowal of the economy" (Bourdieu 1996) through which health officers' economic interests are renounced. By accumulating symbolic capital via mass circumcisions, health officers sought to fashion themselves as carers of the poor, an image that was approved and expected by locals. In doing so, they also aimed to portray other circumcisers as self-interested and greedy.

The act of disavowal in psychoanalysis always goes hand in hand with that of avowal, and thus with the anxiety stemming from the conflict between the two (Laplanche and Pontalis 1988). The commodification of biomedicalized male circumcision proved to be both thrilling and threatening for health officers, who wanted to establish themselves in their new communities where pursuing profits from male circumcision would be frowned upon. They thus bound themselves to the medicalization of the 1960s, which fully monetized performing circumcision through sustaining a balanced distance from monetization. And the too-muchness associated with the position of the rational and calculative subject became especially clear when circumcisers consistently avoided the topic of prices for their services. For instance, one circumciser, as we saw, covered the price of his circumcisions with his hand while showing me the list of the circumcisions he performed for free. For circumcisers, the topic of money was generally a source of embarrassment.

Health officers' ambivalent economic subjectivity emerged from an inegalitarian welfare arrangement combined with the competitive field of male circumcision during the developmentalist era. The same institutional arrangements also generated moral conflicts for circumcisers who competed against each other. Low-income families' lack of control over how their sons were circumcised at mass circumcisions inadvertently created an opportunity for circumcisers to accrue not only symbolic profits in the form of recognition but also cultural capital in the form of skills and, to some extent, economic capital. Yet performing mass circumcision came at the cost of lowering the quality of care provided for the boys at these charity events. Thus, some circumcisers changed the organization of these operations to make it consistent with their moral values.

Mass circumcisions were based on the anonymity of the poor—anonymity that revealed the limits of the developmentalist project's aim to create healthy citizens. The biomedical model drew on the notion of a bounded and isolated body, the suffering of which is assumed to be organic, acute, and internal and capable of being eliminated via surgical instruments and professional skills and knowledge. While this model required that individualized attention and care should be provided for each boy, only the nonpoor typically received this care, as the bodies of the poor were rendered indistinguishable from each other in mass circumcision contexts. Despite its stated claim to overcome inequalities in accessing health care, the health care—more specifically biomedical care—infrastructure of the 1960s reproduced health inequalities in male circumcision.

Although, starting in the 2000s, the neoliberal restructuring of health care services and medicalized male circumcisions sought to rectify these health inequalities, these attempts likewise culminated in generating a new form of inequality in male circumcision, one based on psychological care. The next two chapters examine this new form of inequality and how it has shaped the subjectivities of circumcisers by comparing the two main classed settings where male circumcisions have been performed in recent decades in Turkey.

I was waiting to interview a urologist in a private hospital in an upper-middle-class neighborhood of Istanbul. As usual, I arrived at the hospital earlier than the appointment time, hoping to have a chance to observe and talk to families. I struck up a conversation with a family of two parents and a seven-year-old boy, who were also waiting in the waiting room. Their only child, Emre, had a consultation appointment with the doctor. Fifteen minutes into our conversation, the urologist invited all the family members to his office and talked to them for about ten minutes. Then, Emre came out of the office alone and sat across from me. He was shy, looking at the ground. At one point, he lifted his head, smiled at me, and I smiled back. He then asked, "Will it hurt?"

Fear of male circumcision is widespread in Turkey. During my research, I listened to many stories of adult men who as boys escaped circumcision in villages. Itinerant circumcisers, as described in chapter 1, typically visited a village for circumcision without an appointment and moved to the next one on the same day. Boys could sometimes hide from itinerant circumcisers—only to get circumcised the next summer. Also, some had heard many frightening jokes about circumcision instruments from their peers or from male adults. Or others may have watched a Turkish comedy movie with an insinuation that circumcisers cut penises with an ax. "Does it hurt?" thus becomes the most urgent question boys like Emre ask about male circumcision.

My answer to Emre was short, yet meant to be comforting: "No, don't worry." After his parents came out of the doctor's office, I went in to talk to Dr. Sabit. Dr. Sabit, a senior urologist with decades of experience in male circumcision, had worked at a public hospital before transferring to the private hospital ten years ago. Switching from the public to private sector is not uncommon among senior doctors, as the latter offer higher salaries and better working conditions. I first asked Dr. Sabit about his conversation with Emre. He said that he wanted to inform him of the details of the operation and comfort him. They had a friendly conversation where Dr. Sabit asked Emre some questions about his personal life such as his school performance and his favorite soccer team:

> Communication with children is essential if you want to win their trust. They should not see circumcision as a punishment. A practitioner should know about child psychology. Of course, we are not psychologists, and we cannot do their jobs, but we should act *like* one and prepare boys psychologically. We are paying attention to this more now.

For Dr. Sabit, a safe operation requires more than the use of local anesthesia, sutures, disinfection, and good cutting skills: it should also ensure boys' psychological well-being. A practitioner should consider the prevalence of the fear of circumcision; pay close attention to his interactions with boys and their inner worlds, moods, and behaviors; and establish rapport with them before and during operations.

This chapter examines how and why circumcisers have transformed themselves into *psychologists-by-proxy* in the neoliberal era. During the developmentalist era, health officers used a biomedical model of harm and care, framing circumcision pain as a physical pain to be managed via surgical techniques. They did not see the fear of circumcision as a moral and professional concern of its own, demanding separate actions and techniques, since the use of surgical techniques, they assumed, was sufficient to address fear as well: if local anesthesia could eradicate pain, then why the fear of the operation?

Starting in the 2000s, experts—medical professionals and psychologists—broke away from the biomedical model and came to legitimize fear as a distinct target for surveillance and intervention. They elaborated on a new medical model of harm, a biopsychosocial model, that suggests that harm in male circumcision cannot always be traced to organic and physiological causes, as it can also be psychological, arising from boys' interactions with their surroundings: family, circumcisers, friends, and society at large. This model calls for attention to boys' subjective experience of male circumcision, problematizes certain habits around the operation, and requires that circumcisers (and families) be proactive in sheltering boys from what can cause emotional scars in them.

The chapter argues that circumcisers during the neoliberal era have harnessed the trauma-based model of care, pain, and harm to middle-class consumerism. They reflect morally and scientifically on what constitutes care and harm in male circumcision, attend to boys' inner worlds and environment, and create a spatial arrangement—a strategy of *splitting*—that isolates and separates boys from each other to minimize their exposure to each other's fears. Boys' emotional distress and outbursts in these medical spaces are evaluated by both families and circumcisers as *failures* on the part of the latter—failures that would undermine their professional status. Health professionals thus want to contain boys' fear in order to prevent it from condensing into not only trauma but also customer dissatisfaction.

Although uncertainties concerning medical care in male circumcision have always existed, the biopsychosocial model of pain amplifies those uncertainties, since boys' fear of circumcision can be triggered unexpectedly and their moods and emotions can be unpredictable. In contrast, such uncertainties are incompatible with consumerism, which demands predictable and flawless circumcisions. Circumcisers increasingly face relentless pressure stemming from the conflict between uncertainties and consumerism. Thus, they attach themselves to the position of psychologist-by-proxy only ambivalently: they distance themselves from the position via certain organizational strategies, especially the strategy of splitting. Through this strategy, circumcisers simultaneously avow and disavow the inevitability of uncertainty and seek to make the emotional burden occasioned by consumer fetishism (fetishism that posits consumer satisfaction as the absolute value and supreme criterion for success in health care services) bearable for themselves.

THE BIOPSYCHOSOCIAL MODEL

In recent decades, the biopsychosocial model has gained wide attention in medicine in Turkey and elsewhere, as it is believed to better attend to the complexity of illness experiences than the biomedical model.[1] Medical anthropologists and sociologists had long shown the deficiency of the biomedical model for addressing various forms of pain such as chronic pain and chronic fatigue syndrome.[2] This reductionist model delegitimizes non-acute forms of pain as unreal because no physiological or organic basis of pain can be detected. In contrast, the biopsychosocial model, it is argued, presents a new way of understanding how "suffering, disease, and illness are affected by multiple levels of the organization, from the societal to the molecular" (Borrell-Carrió et al. 2004, p. 576). It highlights social, psychological, and environmental factors as key contributors to the development and experiences of illness and disease— factors irreducible to laws of physiology.

The biopsychosocial model views subjective experience (of both patients and medical professionals) as crucial for diagnoses and health outcomes, emphasizing the importance of cultivating a more participatory clinician-patient relationship based on trust and empathy. Scholars argued that the advantage of the biopsychosocial model over the biomedical model becomes prominent as the reductionist biomedical model often assumes a certain demographic group (for instance, a white middle-class man) to be the normal patient—a type of patient whose health is much less subject to social forces such as racism and sexism than other patients from other groups such as black people and women.[3] Taking such forces into account, as the biopsychosocial model does, can, it is claimed, provide crucial insights into the health-related problems unique to subordinate groups.

In recent decades, health professionals in male circumcision in Turkey have also increasingly been using a biopsychosocial model while seeking to achieve consumer satisfaction and comfort. The middle-class medical settings that this chapter analyzes can be seen as part of the growing service industry in Turkey and elsewhere. Scholars have highlighted the centrality of emotions or affects to this economy by showing how "emotional labor" (Hochschild 2012), "feeling labor" (Korkman 2015a), "affective labor" (Clough 2008), or "aesthetic labor" (Warhurst and Nickson 2007) facilitate the expansion of market norms and conditions of precarity into new areas ranging from retail and hospitality industries to the modeling industry and health care.

I propose "psychological care" as another (emic) concept for capturing the same general dynamics of labor in the service economy. Psychological care consists of health professionals' efforts to attune themselves to even minor deviations and fluctuations in boys' moods and identify, redirect, and contain them before the eruption of full-blown disruptions. Emotions in these settings are seen as objects of management and control as much as fluid, amorphous, and contagious intensities. Psychological care thus refers to both nonconscious (intuitions and embodied knowledge) and conscious (language and performance) dimensions of the techniques used by circumcisers.[4]

Moreover, I suggest that the tension between consumer fetishism and uncertainties as well as the anxiety that derives therefrom are all intrinsic to the service economy. In this economy, service providers often engage in a strategy of splitting similar to the one this chapter discusses: a strategy whereby providers hide or keep in the background the emotions and practices that they think would upset their customers. A psychoanalytically informed understanding of subjectivity as centered on ambivalences can help elucidate the intrapsychic and contradictory dynamics of this labor and the pressure of uncertainties unique to the service economy in general.

In what follows, I focus on the ways in which both the trauma-based psychological model of pain and care and neoliberal consumerism have changed the field of male circumcision. A series of political, discursive, and institutional changes and events have allowed for the rise and expansion of psychology, psychiatry, and consumerism in recent decades in the society of Turkey. And each development has introduced into male circumcision new discrete symbols, language, and metrics of success and worth.

Following the analysis of each development, the last section discusses in depth the convergence between the trauma-based model of care and consumerism in middle-class settings. It highlights the anxiety that practitioners experience in conjunction with the "psy techniques" (Rose 1996)—anxiety that emerges from the tension between inevitable uncertainties concerning care as opposed to consumerism that demands flawless circumcision. I show how managing this tension has been essential to circumcisers' affective investment in their new position as circumcisers who cater to the needs of customers.

TRAUMA

The growing influence of trauma-based discourse on male circumcision should not be isolated from broader changes in mental health policies in Turkey. The historical trajectory of these policies largely paralleled the same development observed in the West: from institutionalization to deinstitutionalization. In Turkey, the institutionalization period dating from the early nineteenth century to the mid-twentieth century saw the first mental health legislation, the establishment of psychiatric hospitals and units across the country, the recognition of psychiatry as a discipline, and reforms in traditional mental asylums (Artvinli 2013; Bilir and Artvinli 2021).

Lasting from the end of World War II to the 1970s, the first wave of deinstitutionalization, "community-based care," began with the implementation of the new outpatient mental health care clinics and psychoactive medications. As part of the health care project of the 1960s, the psychiatrist and chief doctor Faruk Bayülkem initiated a series of education and information campaigns to change the stigmatized language around mental health and communicate to the public scientific knowledge about mental disorders. In Istanbul, an open-door policy was implemented, new mental health dispensaries were opened, and new departments led by professional nurses, social workers, and psychologists became established "for advanced psychiatric rehabilitation and the academic studies of psychiatrists" (Bilir and Artvinli 2021, p. 6). Additionally, small workshops were designated as supportive treatment mechanisms to "ease the discharge of patients from mental hospitals" (Bilir and Artvinli 2021, p. 6). From the 1980s onwards, the ongoing reforms removed patients from mental institutions to reduce the number of inpatients and of psychiatric beds.

Overall, the political and institutional efforts of the early decades of the deinstitutionalization period both incorporated mental health care into the general health system and combined asylums with communities. However, the turning point of the history of deinstitutionalization was the two major earthquakes, commonly referred to as the 1999 Marmara earthquake. These devastating earthquakes claimed more than 17,000 deaths with hundreds of thousands injured, and it displaced and traumatized more than a million people. While revealing the deficiencies of mental health services, the disaster also led to the expansion of the authority of psychiatry in Turkey (Aker et al. 2007), as it "facilitated psychiatry's movement beyond the clinic, as a form of expertise granted new value to speak about the affective, behavioral and political vicissitudes of every day" (Dole 2015, p. 283). In the ensuing days and months, many governmental and nongovernmental organizations and professionals, including psychologists and psychiatrists, flooded the area with assistance, and widespread screenings were performed with the purpose of rehabilitation and treatment (Aker et al. 2007).

Although psychiatric traumatology in Turkey dates back to World War I (Açiksöz 2015), only in the aftermath of the earthquakes did it begin to appear in the political, medical, and academic discourses (Aker et al. 2007; Dole 2015). Mental health professionals working with psychotherapeutic and psychosocial approaches to the treatment of psychological trauma would "gain influence in clinical practice" (Dole 2015, p. 283). The number of studies about psychological trauma doubled, the translation of diagnostic instruments became standardized, and the epidemiological basis of PTSD was established.

In the meantime, trauma has become written into the political and academic language for understanding and contesting different forms of violence, suffering, and human rights violations. Starting in the 2000s, for example, the excavation of past traumas experienced by Kurds, Armenians, Alevis, and leftists was believed to contribute to the democratization of the country as well as the therapeutic healing of these groups. "Coming to terms with the past" discourse sought to rewrite the history of Turkey through the temporality of trauma and privileged "memory as the ultimate key to collective redemption" (Kaya 2015, p. 682). Trauma in Turkey has become a "major signifier" that relates present suffering to past violence and suffering (Fassin 2009).

Moreover, in recent decades psychology and its various subfields (such as developmental psychology) have begun to play a key role in institutional practices. The Turkish military has integrated psychiatry into its screening process for those who request an exemption from compulsory military service (Başaran 2014). Also, counseling services have become an essential component of the school system, providing educational guidance and support for students. Furthermore, the rising number of private universities has stimulated the opening of new psychology departments and increasing enrollment in psychology programs at all levels. The establishment of psychology as a new occupational niche has gone hand in hand with the increasing availability of psychological consultation services for urban and educated middle classes in large cities (Kayaoğlu and Batur 2013).

The influence of psychology in Turkey did not remain within the confines of institutions and has permeated cultural representations and normative ideas about the self and the family that circulate in public. Psychological discourses, knowledge, and concepts (including trauma) have gradually become available to various segments of society via mass media such as television programs, self-help books, magazines, and newspapers. The society of Turkey has become increasingly familiar with psychological vocabularies about various issues, including, but not limited to, intimate relationships (such as child-rearing practices, marriage, love, and sexuality) and mental illnesses and disorders— albeit the reception of psychology across the society varies by such factors as age, class, and gender.

Psychology and psychiatry have shaped male circumcision in two main ways: one is that the opponents of male circumcision now use the idiom of trauma to justify their moral stance against male circumcision. Male circumcision, they argue, causes psychological problems and thus should be ended. Yet, this approach has remained weak and marginalized.

Second, a more mainstream perspective on the relationship between trauma and male circumcision was to adopt the same harm reduction approach observed in the early republican period. As discussed in chapter 2, rather than banning male circumcision, the Turkish ruling elites decided to bring it under medico-bureaucratic authority to manage the potential harm that the operation could cause, with harm solely conceived as physical at that time. Similarly, the adoption of the trauma-based model of pain and care in male circumcision was largely what led to deliberations over how, rather than whether, male circumcision should be performed. Psychologists warned against the potentially traumatic effects of male circumcision, urging families and practitioners to take into account boys' sexual, emotional, and cognitive development in relation to harmful habits concerning male circumcision.

A pressing issue was the question of the appropriate age for male circumcision, which prompted differing answers from experts. Using a popular Freudian language, some claimed that boys between the ages of two and six should not be circumcised, as those boys tend to suffer "castration anxiety." During this period, it was claimed, boys feel scared of their fathers and are more likely to see circumcision as a punishment than they would at a different age.[5] Others have claimed that boys older than the age of seven can be very susceptible to anxious thoughts due to their advanced cognitive development and have therefore recommended against circumcision past that age. Regardless of their opinions about the ideal circumcision age, however, experts have agreed that the parents' role is key to boys' psychological well-being. As clinical child and adolescent psychologist F. Işıl Yenikaynak (2018) says:

> We don't approve frightening jokes about male circumcision. It is inappropriate to say that it would hurt so much or all of it [the penis] would be cut off. Clear and accurate information is important. Saying "it won't hurt at all" is also wrong. Parents should tell their sons that they might feel a little bit of pain. Parents can also try to comfort their kids by buying them toys and organizing a celebration. In the days leading up to the operation, it is important to keep the boys away from their circumcised peers since their peers may talk about the operation in an exaggerated manner. (*Haberler*)

As in the case of the biomedical model of pain, the psychological model charges families with the role of protecting boys from the potential harm that male circumcision can cause. However, families' new role is more open-ended, vague, and demanding than the one entailed by the biomedical model. While parents during the developmentalist era were merely expected to agree to the use of medical techniques and (for mothers, typically) to participate to some extent in the postsurgical care, the trauma-based model of care requires that parents regularly monitor their own behaviors, feelings, and reactions as much as their interactions with their sons. This is so because harm within this model is no longer seen only as organic or physiological.

For the biomedical model, the target of medical intervention was fixed: the penis. To manage the physical pain, all a circumciser needed to do was to inject a local anesthetic into the groin area and suture the incision. With the addition of the psychological model, the object of intervention for safe circumcision proliferated, as fear can in principle arise from anything that surrounds boys, such as words, sounds, silences, gestures, and images. These signs within the new model can no longer be seen as of secondary importance, let alone be dismissed as mere illusions, as the biomedical model would suggest. Parents are thus expected to become preemptive in interacting with their sons, because while incisions on the penis can be sutured, emotional scars can't. Trauma speaks, in some sense, to an irrecoverable loss. It can always already be too late.

The psychological model of harm in male circumcision expects the same from health professionals: constant caution and vigilance concerning boys' inner worlds. At the same time, health professionals also compete for demands for circumcision, therefore feeling pressured to deliver satisfaction and comfort for all family members as well as boys. Before analyzing health professionals' changing practices, a brief digression into a historical account of the rise of the service economy and consumerism in health care is in order. This section will support a better understanding of how the psychological model of pain has been intertwined with neoliberal consumerism in male circumcision in Turkey.

CONSUMERISM

In the post-1980 era, the major developments in Turkey included economic liberalization, the declining power of the leftist opposition (socialist parties and unions), and the rise of Islamist political parties—all made possible by the 1980 coup d'état. The Turkish army took over the executive power in 1980 and suppressed the leftist opposition, closed trade unions, and imprisoned activists (Cosar and Yegenoglu 2009). The coup precluded the possible emergence of strong alternative voices opposing the neoliberal policies unleashed during the coming decades. The military also took the leading role in introducing the private sector into certain public domains. The 1982 constitution, ratified by popular referendum under military rule (1980–1983), emphasized the regulatory role of the state and, for the first time, the importance of the private sector as an actor in health care (Günal 2008).

The end of the military rule in 1983 heralded the revival of electoral democracy and the acceleration of economic liberalization overseen by the IMF and the World Bank. The successive single-party and coalition governments moved the economy from import substitution developmentalism to liberal, export-driven growth by lifting many protectionist measures, privatizing public enterprises, and facilitating the intrusion of multinational companies and a dizzying influx of imported luxury goods to the market. The internationalization of retail trade and services by means of high-street brands and the increasing number of new shopping venues (for instance, exclusive boutiques and large shopping malls catering to a wider clientele) began to change the daily lives of urbanites across social classes in diverse ways.

Moreover, with the breaking of the state monopoly over mass media and the proliferation of private television channels in the early 1990s and more recent decades, the internet and social media have multiplied people's encounters with commodity images embodying the promises of secular salvation, prosperity, immediate gratification, and progress through pleasure. Society-wide consumerism has brought forth new axes of social differentiation and stratification, "precipitating both a greater fragmentation of social identities and an increasing complexity in their public articulation" (Kandiyoti and Saktanber 2002, 5). Consumption began to shape and redefine identities, introducing Western-style consumerism as a marker of middle-class status, emergent subcultural expressions among the youth, and the commodification of both secular and Islamic symbols in public, to name a few (Navaro-Yashin 2002b; Özyürek 2006).

The rise of consumerism in Turkey has reinforced what we can call the "sovereign consumer,"[6] a self-positing fantasy intrinsic to the market fundamentalism that views the market as a site of salvation and prosperity. The figure of the sovereign consumer refers to a self-sufficient, self-contained, and infallible ideal animated in the desire for immediacy ("this is what customers want"), epistemic naivety ("well-informed consumers"), and moral absolutism ("the customer is always right"). More specifically, it signifies an autonomous and self-identical subject who (supposedly) knows what is best for them, who is the sole arbiter of market competition, and thus whose choices steer the market.

The sovereign consumer is a powerful fiction that not only has driven government policies since the 1980s on a macro level across countries but also has become a major site of identifications, fantasies, and attachments.[7] And as evidenced by its presence across class settings, it entertains the idea of relative autonomy from the economic conditions requisite for its full materialization (as discussed in chapter 5, the same fiction can feel disappointing for those who cannot meet these conditions), as it legitimizes boundaries and hierarchies between actors, crowds out nonmarket incentives, and perpetuates the drive for consumption.

In recent decades, health professionals' circumcision practices have been shaped by the paired goals of providing psychological care and sustaining the sovereign consumer—the consumer who expects an enjoyable and memorable circumcision event where emotional discomfort and outbursts are minimized, if not eliminated. Before closely analyzing the relationship between the trauma-based model of harm and care and consumerism, two concepts should be clarified. First, just as the health officers' claim that physical pain was not much of a concern in circumcisions performed by itinerant circumcisers was, as chapter 1 demonstrated, false, it is important to avoid assuming that the rise of the trauma-based model was preceded by an absence of concern or worry regarding fear in male circumcision. Male circumcision had always been a feared practice, and it would be wrong to claim that families and circumcisers had never attended to the fear of circumcision in the past. That said, this chapter claims, not until a few decades ago did fear of circumcision become a distinct object of systematic and calculated deliberations, practices, and strategies on the part of practitioners.

Second, the previous chapters use the term "market" to describe the competition between circumcisers for the demands for male circumcision during the developmentalist era. However, the difference between these two periods can't be overstated: while the circumcision market of the 1960s was a *byproduct* of state intervention as health officers used their official capacity for personal financial gains, the AKP's neoliberalism has purposefully turned the market—its symbols, values, and metrics of success—into an explicit guide for policies, a solution for social problems, and a route for happiness and satisfaction in areas including health care in general and male circumcision in particular. In part, thus, I am interested in the question of how the field of male circumcision has been remade in the image of the market and the kind of subjectivity this transformation requires.

COMMUNICATION

In a southern town, I interviewed Salim, a sixty-five-year-old health officer with forty years of experience in male circumcision. We first started chatting outside his home and then he kindly invited me into his home to avoid the scorching sun on what was a typically hot August day for that region. As Sünnetçi Salim was taking his circumcision instruments from his bag one by one and explaining them, I was taking sips of the fresh homemade lemonade his wife, Selma, had made. I asked about Sünnetçi Salim's relationships with locals:

AUTHOR: Did locals like your circumcision style when you first started?
SALİM: Yes, they did. I have an advantage, though. I also go to families' homes for vaccination. Kids have seen their uncle Salim since birth. They see me as not a circumciser but rather a health professional, someone who can do good for them. I also talk to boys before the operation to appease their fear of the circumciser.
SELMA: There is no house around here that Salim has not already visited. People know him and trust him.
SALİM: Eighty percent of circumcision is about psychology. Then, comes asepsis and antisepsis. The unconscious is very important. A boy's trauma stemming from his childhood and his relationship with his mother and father can come to the surface. I talk to children, give them candies or Turkish delight and inform them of the steps of circumcision. I show them the instruments, and if I am using chloroethyl spray for local anesthesia, I first spray it on their hands. I prepare them for circumcision by talking to them and telling them that there is nothing to be afraid of. That is the most important part. Cutting the foreskin off properly is not the most important part of circumcision. That is what the law requires anyways. That's the physical part. More importantly, you should not cause trauma in the boy.

Sünnetçi Salim was aware that the sünnetçi is a frightening figure for boys in Turkey and that his other professional roles could offset the possible unpleasant effects of his ominous presence in their lives. For operations, he wanted to make sure that boys would know what to expect from him and the procedure and would not, for instance, get startled by the cold feeling of the spray on their penises. These precautions could, he believed, make boys feel safe and in control, preventing their childhood issues suppressed in the unconscious from emerging. Sünnetçi Salim thought that circumcisers should go beyond what the "law" (the 1928 law) requires them to do—that is, biomedical care. For him, psychology had raised the standards for safe circumcision: circumcision should now be considered safe when performed without not only pain and blood but also fear and trauma. It also changed what it means to be a good circumciser: a good circumciser should be self-reflective, as his words, demeanors, and interactions with boys have, Sünnetçi Salim thought, major impacts on boys' mood, fear, and overall well-being.

Over the last two decades, specialists at hospitals and senior health officers like Sünnetçi Salim have been highlighting the importance of psychological care for safe male circumcision. They see *communication* as a key component of this care, because it gives boys an opportunity to ask questions about the operation and express their fears (if any) instead of bottling them up. Communication, in their views, should continue during operations as well. However, a boy's age can sometimes be an obstacle to utilizing this strategy to its fullest potential. Dr. Kapucu, a specialist in his thirties, brought up this issue:

AUTHOR: How do you communicate with boys?
DR. KAPUCU: We explain the operation to those with whom we can communicate. If boys are younger than, let's say, nine, communication gets a bit more difficult. However, regardless of age, if they are too nervous and restless, we hold them down by legs and hands and then circumcise them.
AUTHOR: If you can communicate with them, what do you say?
DR. KAPUCU: We tell them that we will apply an anesthetic and the injection will be small. We show them where we will inject it, and we say that we will then clean the foreskin and they won't feel pain. So, we tell them everything.

Dr. Kapucu had been performing circumcision for several years at a private hospital in a middle-class neighborhood in Istanbul. He carries out the procedures in a room decorated with toys, posters, and garlands, all intended to make boys and their families feel at home. In his conversation with boys, Kapucu mentions the size of injections he uses, because one of the circumcision-related jokes boys often hear in Turkey is that circumcisers use big injections. Yet, when his communication skills fail to generate the desired outcomes, he resorts to force and has boys pinned down to make sure that the operations will not lead to any physical injury to the boys or him. For him, comforting boys and keeping them calm are, in other words, essential to not only their psychological but also their physical well-being.

One can contend that communication with patients is a routine and mundane part of medical operations and that calling it a new practice, as I do, is an overstatement. After all, doctors are expected to provide their patients with information concerning all surgeries. However, it should be emphasized that circumcisers' deliberately crafted sensitivity toward boys' inner lives has grown only with the influence of the trauma-based model in recent decades and that the newness of communication as a skill in male circumcision is evident in senior health professionals' accounts of the changes in their practices.

Fenni Sünnetçi Yunus had been performing circumcision since 1978 or '79 (he could not remember the exact year). I interviewed him at his clinic,[8] and I asked him about the difficulties of the profession:

YUNUS: The biggest problem for us begins in cases where boys are seven years old. Since those boys are very aware of their surroundings, they are more afraid of circumcision than younger boys are. And you know, in Turkey people make jokes about circumcision—like, cutting the penis off with an ax. Since the child at that age cannot tell whether it is real or a joke, he buries all these jokes in his unconscious [bilinçdışı], and when the time comes for circumcision, everything in his unconscious comes out. So, who is going to step in at that moment? The circumciser and his team step in. They operate with the knowledge of the psychological state of the boy and approach the boy in a sensitive manner.

AUTHOR: I noticed that you also talk to boys and try to comfort them before and during the operation. The boys did not even realize that they were being circumcised. Have you always been doing this?

YUNUS: No! How could we know children's world?—I mean, this much child psychology.

AUTHOR: When did you start it then?

YUNUS: When I hold a boy's wrist, I sense what he feels and how he will behave.

AUTHOR: How did this happen though?

YUNUS: Experience. You learn it on the job [bire bir yaşayarak].

Instead of describing a radical break with the past, Sünnetçi Yunus underlined a combination of experiential knowledge with formal and theoretical knowledge concerning child psychology. He claimed to be able to feel a boy's emotional status by holding his wrist, an ability he had developed over the years. Yet, talking to boys before and during the operation became part of his routine practice only after he encountered child psychology as a public and scientific discourse. He highlighted a disturbing ambiguity boys face when exposed to jokes about male circumcision: they can't tell whether it is true that their penises will be cut off with an ax. Using Freudian language, he suggested that boys find this kind of ambiguity too unbearable, suppress it, and then act out before or during the operation. He prided himself and his team on anticipating such acts and managing the boys' unconscious thoughts and feelings.

The impact of psychology on circumcisers also becomes clear in their deliberations over the appropriate age for circumcision. Health professionals—like Drs. Kapucu and Sabit and Fenni Sünnetçi Yunus—now pay more attention to boys' ages, and while some prefer circumcising boys who, they believe, are old enough to communicate effectively with adults, others would rather circumcise younger boys, as older boys tend to feel more anxious about the operation. A few circumcisers even go so far as to turn down families with sons around the age of three or four and recommend against circumcision until their sons get older. As health officer Eryar said:

> Families sometimes listen to us and bring their sons back when they are seven or eight years old. Look, we are not in this business for money. If a boy is two years old, he will cry no matter what. Even if we don't hurt him. He will cry. If you look at a three-year-old boy, his hand is always on his crotch, his interest is in that area. An older boy, a seven- or eight-year-old boy, can better communicate with their parents after the operation. If they are in pain or it feels itchy or needs to pee, they can tell it to their mothers. If families want their sons to have a good memory of their circumcisions, then what is the point in doing it when they are three years old? Those kids are not going to remember it as a happy event, right?

If male circumcision is a milestone in a boy's life, an event to be remembered fondly in the future, then families, Sünnetçi Eryar argued, should wait until their sons are mature enough emotionally and cognitively. Sünnetçi Eryar did not trust his communication skills with boys as young as two years old, who, in his view, couldn't properly express their emotions to adults. Words would be replaced by cries and tantrums, he added. In contrast, older boys can enjoy their circumcisions without feeling the urge to protect their penises.

The deliberations over the relationship between age and psychology included neonatal circumcisions, as well. Neonatal circumcisions are typically performed by doctors at hospitals and have in recent decades become a viable alternative to regular circumcisions in Turkey. This type of circumcision particularly appeals to educated middle- and upper-middle-class urban families who either have no interest in the ritualistic or religious aspect of the practice or have a plan to organize a celebration in the future. Compared to regular circumcision, infant circumcision is claimed to have a shorter recovery period and pose lower risks for postoperative complications. Some health professionals add that infants feel only a minor discomfort (if any) due to their pain threshold being higher than older children's. In my conversation with Saygun, a urologist in his fifties, we discussed neonatal circumcision in relation to trauma:

AUTHOR: Do you also perform neonatal circumcision?
SAYGUN: Yes, I do. Families are now concerned about the psychological effects of circumcision on their children. The fact that the fear of circumcision becomes more intense for cognitively developed kids makes parents worry. The questions of how to prepare children for circumcision and to protect them from its psychological effects begin to puzzle parents. They either make up excuses to postpone the circumcision or take a risk by having their sons circumcised under general anesthesia. But I think the only solution to eliminate or at least minimize traumatic experience is neonatal circumcision.

Saygun supports neonatal circumcisions for being less harmful than regular circumcisions, highlighting a vicious circle: boys at regular circumcisions know that they will be circumcised, even though they might not know when, and are often overwhelmed by distressing thoughts. And sons' worries then feed parents' worries, and so on. Thus, neonatal circumcision is, for Saygun, an ideal solution to the dread experienced by all members of the family in relation to male circumcision.

Such concerns and deliberations about the proper circumcision age should be seen as part of health professionals' overall efforts to find clear indicators of fear of male circumcision, as well as a concrete guide of action to anticipate and manage this fear. However, health professionals' conflicting views on the issue show how elusive, uncontrollable, and unpredictable the fear of male circumcision can be. Fear of circumcision as an object of control generates greater uncertainties and risks of failure for health professionals than does physical pain. As previous chapters mention, health officers and itinerant circumcisers have confronted uncertainties concerning the safety of the operations, especially when they first began to perform circumcision in the 1960s. "What if it bleeds overnight?" and "What if I cut it too much?" were some of the troubling questions that often cost them sleep. Sometimes, their nightmares almost came true. Sünnetçi Faruk shared a story about overweight boys that I also heard from a few other health officers:

Once, I got a call at midnight from a family whose son I circumcised that day. They said, "His penis is gone." I said, "What do you mean 'it is gone'?" "We can't see it," they said. I was young and panicked a lot. I went straight to their house and saw the family surrounding the boy. They all looked very sad, which made me even more worried. I checked the boy's penis and indeed could not see it [he smiles]. The boy was overweight, and I realized that his penis was retracted. I then popped it back up [he smiles again].

Such uncertainties, risks, and doubts were at times so overwhelming that some health officers and some itinerant circumcisers' sons never started performing circumcision. That said, the nature of problems that worried circumcisers in the past was mainly physical (for instance, bleeding), and their causes were few and well known, such as cutting the foreskin improperly. The senior circumcisers who mentioned this added that their concerns abated, though they may not have completely disappeared, as they gained more experience.

When dealing with the fear of circumcision, however, circumcisers faced a different and more difficult situation as uncertainties concerning the care, harm, and responsibility increased in range, depth, and frequency. This is so because erratic changes in moods can occur without a clear warning signal, making circumcisers wonder: Is he going to cry? Why does he look upset? Is it something I said? Is it the scalpel blade I am holding? Is it the other kid who is crying? Parents concerned about their sons' psychological well-being want to see their sons' happy faces before, during, and after the operation. However, a happy face can turn into a sad one for countless reasons. Fear of circumcision is hard to control. And it is contagious.

There are, of course, some common culprits of this fear, such as the circumciser and the circumcision instruments, and, as we saw, practitioners try to change how boys perceive these two presences by communicating with them in a soothing voice and explaining the instruments. In doing so, they seek to induce specific sensations in boys, such as calmness, and neutralize their fear. Yet uncertainties around fear of circumcision and the pressure to perform flawless procedures became so intense that circumcisers also introduced a new organizational infrastructure.

ATMOSPHERE

Private hospitals and private clinics run by senior health officers were until very recently the main service providers of male circumcision in large cities. Health officers at these clinics offered a variety of services: preparing and applying injections, dressing wounds, measuring blood pressure, providing first aid, and male circumcision. And some of them who serve middle-class clienteles focused solely on circumcision have competed against private hospitals and prided themselves on providing not only a hospital-like environment for families but also what hospitals, they claimed, cannot offer: a "traditional" and "warmer" circumcision experience. A welcome sign at one private clinic reads:

> Our clinic performs only circumcisions and is different from ordinary hospitals. It is designed so that boys are circumcised without being aware of the operation, in an entertaining way. Indeed, our staff is trained to provide such comfort for children and families . . . our clinic makes a difference and distinguishes itself from others by turning circumcisions into entertainment where boys have no fear of circumcision. Our clinic is taken as a model by our competitors and has become a brand itself . . . we are honored to host our valued guests and friends.

This clinic has been run by Fenni Sünnetçi Yunus (whom I mentioned earlier) since 1989. Sünnetçi Yunus learned the practice during his mandatory military service at a military hospital. There, he assisted surgeons with circumcisions and was also taught by senior nurses how to dress a wound and administer injections. He performed a few procedures at the hospital, too. By the end of his military service, he received a license from the military hospital for performing minor medical tasks, including male circumcision, in his civilian life.

Over the course of my research, I frequented his one-floor clinic, which is located on the fourth floor of a building in Istanbul. During my first visit, I was told that Sünnetçi Yunus was performing an operation and I should wait in the waiting room with the other families. The room was well decorated and had a small area for toys and games. Sünnetçi Yunus was inside the operating room with the door closed behind him. In the meantime, other boys were playing games and waiting for their turns while their family members (parents and grandparents) were sitting and chatting on leather chairs. As I was glancing around the room, a staff member suddenly began to play very loud music. Was the music for the boy inside the operating room, who was now circumcised and ready to come out for his celebration? I kept my eyes on the door, but no one came out. The music stopped after a few minutes, and it seemed like I was the only one in the waiting room who was puzzled by it.

I was then called by Sünnetçi Yunus's assistant into the operating room for the interview. At first glance, the operating room, which was also his office, consisted of what one would expect from a standard operating room and office: an operating table, surgical instruments, a desk, a desk computer, and Sünnetçi Yunus's license on a wall. As I continued looking around, I was surprised to see a TV screen facing the operating table and a PlayStation remote controller on the side of the table. Sünnetçi Yunus and I then sat down for the interview. I was eager to ask him about the PlayStation and the loud music. Yet, before I could ask him any question, a staff member walked in to inform Sünnetçi Yunus that the next boy was ready for circumcision. Yunus and I stepped outside the room: he greeted the boy and put his arm around him as the same staff member handed him a microphone. The following conversation transpired between Sünnetçi Yunus and the boy:

YUNUS: What is your name?
THE BOY: Murat Yaman.
YUNUS: How old are you?
MURAT: Seven.
YUNUS: When are you going to be circumcised?
MURAT: Today.
YUNUS: No, not today. Tomorrow. Today we will only put two different kinds of cream; one is banana-flavored and the other one is lemon-flavored. You will play PlayStation inside the room and collect points. Okay?
MURAT: Okay.
YUNUS: Now I am going to ask you a few questions. Who is the most beautiful girl in your class?
MURAT: Nisa (he smiles).
YUNUS: What (soccer) team are you supporting?
MURAT: Fener.
YUNUS: Fener? Everyone is supporting Fener! Anyways, now repeat after me: I pledge on my honor to be a man.
MURAT: I pledge on my honor to be a man.
YUNUS: Never break my word.
MURAT: Never break my word.
YUNUS: Always support Fener.
MURAT: Always support Fener.
YUNUS: Good job!

Murat was prompted by Sünnetçi Yunus to perform a dominant script of masculinity in Turkey that links male circumcision to other practices of masculinity. Breaking your word signals weakness in men—for instance, you can be called an "ibne" (fag)—and being a soccer team fan serves as a heterosexual male-bonding practice. Changing your favorite team can be compared to religious conversion, which is highly frowned upon in Turkey. It can also make you seem less of a man and turn you into a target for ridicule.

After the initial performance, Murat was taken to the operating room, where he was placed on the operating table for circumcision. I also went in, with others, including his parents, Sünnetçi Yunus, and his assistant. Sünnetçi Yunus turned on the TV screen and the PlayStation, and Murat began to play a game. As he was circumcising Murat, Yunus struck up a casual conversation with him. He dared Murat to collect a certain number of points at the game and congratulated him for each point he gained. In doing so, Sünnetçi Yunus was trying to keep Murat distracted.

As Yunus was about to cut off the foreskin, his assistant asked the other staff member to play music, which solved my other puzzle as well: the timing of the music showed that it was meant to drown out the voice of boys in the operating room in case they screamed or cried. Sünnetçi Yunus was certainly worried about Murat's psychological well-being, as he was doing his best to keep Murat calm and comfortable. However, he knew that his efforts could not guarantee that Murat would not cry for some reason that Sünnetçi Yunus could not anticipate. He also knew that fear of male circumcision is contagious: if Murat cried, the boys in the waiting room could hear him and become anxious too.

Not only did Murat not cry during the operation, but he wasn't even aware of his foreskin being cut off as he was intensely focused on the game. In the meantime, another staff member was taking a video of the operation (and the rest of the event), which later became available for Murat's family to purchase. Once Yunus completed the operation, we all stepped outside of the room. Yunus was again handed the microphone, standing in front of the other families in the waiting room:

YUNUS: Murat, you are now a man. You were very brave. You did not cry. I congratulate you on your courage. So, Murat, tell us, did it hurt?
MURAT: No.
YUNUS: Bravo, bravo! I hope you will be as brave and successful for the rest of your life as you were here. Here is your "Certificate of Bravery" (Cesaret Belgesi).
MURAT: Thank you.

In the post-operation performance, Sünnetçi Yunus wanted to signal to Murat's family and other families as well that he had completed the circumcision without causing any pain or fear. But even if Murat had felt pain or fear and expressed it somehow in the operating room, the cheerful music would have muffled what could otherwise have been a frightening noise for the other boys and their families in the waiting room. Overall, Sünnetçi Yunus aimed to generate an atmosphere purged of potentially unpleasant or distressing verbal, visual, and sonic effects that might spur fear in boys. After completing Murat's ceremony, the circumciser moved on to the next circumcision and carried out the same performance.

Sünnetçi Yunus wanted to provide both physical and psychological care for boys and transform male circumcision into an enjoyable event for families. His clinic provided not only a visible wall, the door of the operating room, but also an invisible wall, the cheerful music. And both walls separated boys from each other and created a split between what can and should be seen, heard, and said and what cannot and should not—a split through which Sünnetçi Yunus sustained the image of good circumciser who can deliver circumcisions without emotional discomfort or outbursts.

For the same purpose, another clinic used an even more sophisticated strategy. This clinic was located in an upper-middle-class neighborhood in Istanbul and was run by two brothers: health officer Gökçe and urologist Fırat, who also officially owned the clinic. In our conversations, both Gökçe and Fırat highlighted that they did not view circumcision as "some sort of a burden" that boys should forget about or get over with but rather a day for boys to feel special, one that they should remember warmly. As a routine practice, they recommend that parents bring their children to the clinic before scheduling circumcisions so that they could watch how a standard circumcision takes place. Sünnetçi Fırat strongly emphasized the importance of this visit since it, he believes, enables boys to gain familiarity with the procedure and prepare themselves emotionally. "Circumcisions can be traumatic if boys do not know what to expect," he added. The preoperative visits represent another safeguard to make male circumcision more predictable for boys so that they can feel in control and secure. The visits can also help demonstrate the clinic's high-quality services to families as consumers. Consumer satisfaction and boys' well-being are thus inextricably linked to each other.

The clinic typically combines five or six circumcisions, gathering a group of boys and their extended families (sometimes up to fifty people) to boost the joyful atmosphere of the event. The first segment of the performance takes place in a large room with tables and chairs placed in front of a stage. The stage has five tall, red, throne-like chairs and a piano, and the performance starts with the cheerful appearance of a clown with a microphone. With a loud jingle in the background, the clown jumps around on the stage, welcomes the families, and tries to uplift their mood. He then ushers the boys to the stage and lines them up, facing the audience, and asks each of them: What is your name? What soccer team are you a fan of?

After the boys' responses, a singer joins the clown and asks the boys to step down from the stage and join their mothers for a slow dance.[9] This pre-operation ritual reenacts the cultural script of male circumcision as a rite of passage that (supposedly) separates boys from their mothers in their journey to be a man on a symbolic level. As the dance finishes, the boys and their mothers are seated separately again, and Sünnetçi Fırat appears on the stage. Unlike Sünnetçi Yunus, Sünnetçi Fırat recommends full disclosure and does not hide from boys that they are about to be circumcised. He comforts the boys, shows them the instruments he will use, and walks them through the operation. He then begins to apply a local anesthetic to each boy, with the boys' favorite soccer teams' theme songs playing in the background.

In the meantime, the singer invites elderly family members such as parents, grandparents, aunts, and uncles to dance together. Once the local anesthesia takes effect, the music stops, and the singer asks the audience to be quiet. An imam wearing a floor-length vest and a cap then walks solemnly onto the stage. His slow pace fills the formerly uplifting and joyous atmosphere with sobriety and calmness. Women, if not already veiled, cover their hair with kerchiefs distributed by the staff, and as the imam takes a seat and starts praying, everyone raises both their hands up to chest level with the palms facing inside and prays together.

After the praying, the circumciser calls each boy, one by one, and starts the operation while the imam chants, "Allahu Akbar" (Allah is the Greatest). Each boy then disappears from sight and goes into a back room. After ten minutes, they come back to the stage. Following the operation, the clown hands each boy a certificate of manhood and asks them to give a soldier salute, alluding to their next rite of passage—that is, military service.[10] At the same time, the clown recites the well-known expression about male circumcision "Oldu da bitti maşallah, damat olur inşallah" (it has happened at once, may Allah preserve him; he will be a groom, by Allah's will), except he replaces the word "groom" with such occupations as "scientist," "prime minister," and "professor"—occupations aligned with families' cultural capital. Families and the boys then reunite on the stage and dance together again to uplifting music.

When I first watched this performance, I was confused as to why Sünnetçi Fırat sent the boys to another room in the back and then had them back on the stage again. I later found out that in a small room with an operating table and medical equipment the other circumciser, Gökçe, finishes the circumcisions that Fırat begins on the stage. They said that in recent decades they had been carrying out the operations in two phases to be able to manage difficult cases: if a boy cries, then he can be immediately taken to the other room, out of sight. And even if no boy cries, this strategy nonetheless lessens the risk of the audience's exposure to unpleasant scenes, as it shortens the total time that boys spend on the stage. The exact moment a boy could cry is unpredictable. Hence the precaution.

Once I was chatting with Sünnetçi Fırat right before he stepped onto the stage to circumcise boys. I noticed how carefully and anxiously he was watching the performance, always keeping his eyes on the stage. Boys were standing next to each other, facing the audience. One boy looked very upset and scared, which caught Sünnetçi Fırat's attention. He immediately interrupted me: "Hold on, I have to take that kid to the back room. He looks like he will cry. I don't want other kids to see it." He indeed rushed to the stage and then ushered the boy to the other room, and the boy's parents joined them as well. Sünnetçi Gökçe then circumcised the boy after he explained to him the procedure, his parents holding his hand and comforting him. Families watch the first phase of their sons' operations and sometimes take photos of or even film them.

The clinic wanted to provide both biomedical and psychological care for boys without completely divorcing the operation from the rest of the ritual. That said, the circumcisers were also wary of the failures risked in this performance—failures that could give the impression that the circumcisers were not delivering proper psychological care. Any sign of anxiety in boys would thus generate anxiety in circumcisers, an unconscious transmission that can explain why the close and detailed supervision of boys went beyond the relatively public space of the stage at the clinic. On many occasions, when one of the circumcisers or a staff member noticed a boy in the waiting room who looked upset and was about to cry, they would rush to either pull him aside and comfort him inside the room or take him out of the room. They were constantly on alert for possible disruptions of ordinary life at the clinic.

Other clinics also used similar but less sophisticated strategies. I visited Sünnetçi Hikmet's clinic a few times during my research. Once, before an operation, Sünnetçi Hikmet proudly asked me to take photos of his clinic and instruments. He asked the boy to lie on the operating table and had his parents stand by his side. Sünnetçi Hikmet asked the family waiting in the waiting room to step outside. As he was cutting off the boy's foreskin, the boy started crying and Hikmet got panicked and turned to me: "Don't take photos anymore" (I had already put my camera aside). Later, I would find out that sending families in the waiting room outside the clinic was a strategy that Sünnetçi Hikmet routinely used during circumcisions. "I don't want other kids to be scared," he said.

All of these clinics carry out circumcisions based on the assumption of a self that is porous and malleable. Fear of circumcision is seen as not only subjective but also contagious: it refers to both a particular state of the inner world and an affect that moves across bodies, displacing the distinction between the inside and the outside. Health professionals at these clinics persistently, even obsessively, try to identify, interpret, and isolate various indications of fear of male circumcision in faces, voices, words, remarks, and bodily gestures. By controlling visitors' interactions and the circulation of verbal, visual, and sonic images, they aim to filter out the external influences and create a pleasant atmosphere for families.

UNCERTAINTIES

Medical sociologists have written extensively about the emotional, moral, and existential consequences of medical uncertainties for medical professionals. On the one hand, the uncertainties concerning diagnosis, treatment, and prognosis are claimed to be grounded in indeterminacies of knowledge (such as an incomplete mastery of available knowledge and limitations in current knowledge) that will always be present, no matter how great the investment in medical research and information technology (Fox 1980; Light 1979; Reich 2014). Considering that "certainty serves purposes of maintaining professional power and control" (Katz 1984, p. 42), it is unsurprising that medical professionals concern themselves with managing uncertainties via various strategies such as specialization, conformity, dogmatism, and limiting learning to relevant knowledge (Katz 1984; Timmermans and Angell 2001).

On the other hand, scholars have also shown that a degree of uncertainty and its concomitant characteristics such as risk, error, unpredictability, and doubts are not only inevitable but also at times essential to knowing and acting in health care settings. Dismissing or repressing uncertainty can thus produce negative consequences for medical care (Jerak-Zuiderent 2012; Mol 2008). For example, giving equal attention to every nonurgent patient to "avoid the risk that some of them may in fact be in potential danger, would itself introduce risks of less safe care given to obviously urgent patients" (Jerak-Zuiderent 2012, p. 744). As another example, the process of diagnosing a disease initially requires an acknowledgment that the diagnosis is unclear and that only time and treatment can confirm in retrospect whether or not the diagnosis was correct. Therefore, cultivating a capacity for living with uncertainty and allowing for a margin for error can sustain safe medical practices (Jerak-Zuiderent 2012). Ultimately, uncertainties in medical practice are not only inevitable but also sometimes desirable.

This chapter has shown that consumerism in male circumcision is at odds with cultivating such a capacity for tolerating uncertainty, as it demands flawless circumcisions and tends to cast every error, ambiguity, and disruption—namely, bodily expressions of fear in boys—into a sign of inadequacy, failure, and ineptness on the part of practitioners. Circumcisers at the clinics were committed to the new normative understanding of a competent circumciser:

a circumciser attentive to boys' psychology. Yet, they could bind themselves to the position of psychologist-by-proxy only by both disavowing and avowing the inevitability of uncertainties, via spatial and temporary splitting that creates visible and invisible walls—walls that separate what should be seen, heard, and said from what should not. In doing so, they were simultaneously drawn into the biopsychosocial model of pain and harm, and yet they were also defensive against it, as the model multiplied uncertainties that are incompatible with consumerism. These clinics are organized on the implicit assumption that flawless circumcisions are impossible to achieve, as they seek preemptively to incorporate failure into their organizations as a way of defending it against the overwhelming pressure of the fiction of the sovereign consumer—the pressure that circumcisers feel viscerally, as we saw in Sünnetçi Fırat's anxious fixation on the boys on the stage.

My interviewees at times articulated this inevitability explicitly and em-phasized to me a more realistic approach toward their practice than the logic of consumerism would allow. They highlighted that they did their best to provide adequate care for boys, but also, without invoking any stereotype, they added that children are different from each other, with different personalities, interests, and abilities. Some boys are, they said, shier than others. Or they stressed that children's moods, like everyone else's, can change from one day to another, which makes it hard to predict who might be about to cry and make other boys anxious as well. They thus felt like they were asked to accomplish more than what was possible.

These clinics serve middle- and upper-middle-class families. The ordinary life at the clinics was well ordered, without much disruption. When disruptions occurred, they were minor, brief, and containable. What happens when these disruptions become a permanent part of ordinary life itself? How do health professionals and families cope with the perpetual reminder that they both fail to provide adequate care for boys? To answer these questions, the next chapter turns once again to mass circumcision organizations for low-income families.

Chapter 3 discusses how health officers during the developmentalist era viewed mass circumcisions as an opportunity to accumulate (mainly) symbolic profits from the bodies of the poor. They often rushed circumcision procedures in order to perform a vast number of them in a very short time, frequently in unhygienic settings and without proper pre- and postsurgical care such as the sterilization of instruments. Starting in the 2000s, hospital-based mass circumcisions emerged as a response to the infrastructural shortcomings of the mass circumcisions of the developmentalist era. Health authorities, hospital managers, and doctors have gradually aligned with efforts to move the venues of mass circumcisions from non-medical settings under the authority of health officers to hospitals under the authority of doctors.

This chapter discusses the emergence and consequences of hospital-based mass circumcisions by analyzing health professionals' moral dilemmas concerning the operations. Today, health professionals at both private and public hospitals are influenced by the trauma-based model of care in male circumcision. However, as we shall see, those who perform mass circumcisions in low-ranking private hospitals fall short of delivering what they consider proper care, especially psychological care, due to difficult working conditions such as overcrowded hospital floors and the shortage of time available for each patient. These doctors are afflicted with an ongoing burden of failure.

The chapter argues that doctors project this burden onto two ideological figures: Deceitful Child and Bad Parents. While the former rests upon biomedical reductionism that delegitimizes boys' psychological suffering, the latter, informed by the stigmatization of the poor in the neoliberal era, acknowledges this suffering and places the blame on low-income families who supposedly have no regard for safe circumcisions. Doctors, via these ideological figures, confront the pressure stemming from the moral imperative of providing psychological care under unfavorable conditions. In doing so, they continue to attach themselves ambivalently to the position of psychologist-by-proxy without assuming the responsibility that this identification calls forth.

In what follows, I first explain the rise of hospital-based mass circumcisions and how doctors and hospitals, as the newcomers to the field, have over the last three decades delegitimized health officers and nonmedical settings as safe for circumcision. I then examine the institutional and organizational changes that have channeled mass operations toward private hospitals and doctors. The remainder of the chapter focuses on the way mass circumcisions are performed at the hospitals in rural-to-urban migrant neighborhoods of large cities, compares it to circumcisions in middle-class settings, and analyzes how health professionals navigate the ethical and professional challenges produced by the persistent infrastructural deficiencies of mass circumcisions in the neoliberal era.

PRIVATE HOSPITALS

In recent decades, hospitals in Turkey, especially private hospitals in large cities, have increasingly performed both individual and mass circumcisions. As the previous chapters show, whereas in the past the beneficiaries of public insurance schemes could have had their sons circumcised at medical institutions, they largely preferred homes because they did not want to separate the operations from the rest of the ritual. That the operation itself was embedded within kinship and neighborly networks was also aligned with the interests of health officers, who wanted to keep their business activities off the book.

In the 2000s, the field of male circumcision began to undergo a major transformation. As part of the health care reform, the AKP (Justice and Development Party) government sought to attract private investments in health care services via subsidies for the private sector—the sector that had been lobbying for further commodification of health care services (Yılmaz 2017). Accordingly, between 2002 and 2015 the number of private hospitals increased from 271 to 562 and the number of beds in private institutions increased from 12,387 to 43,645 (Ministry of Health 2014). Between 2009 and 2017, the private provider sector has grown significantly, undertaking 1.6 million operations per year, which is 34 percent of all surgeries, and performing 53 percent of most complex surgeries. Between 2002 and 2010, the number of minor surgeries, including male circumcision, performed at private hospitals went up from 54,975 to 615,745 per year (Ministry of Health 2008, 2010). In 2015, the top 5 hospital chains made up 13 percent of private hospitals.[1] Public-private partnerships (PPPs) provided the conditions to entice hospital chains to build and operate new facilities by ensuring generous debt assumption undertakings wherein the government committed to taking on the debt of the private partners.

When the private sector began to expand its influence in health care services, male circumcision had already proven to be economically lucrative. Health officers had maintained control over their private practices for decades without much challenge from other medical professionals. Doctors, as my interviewees mentioned, have tended to view male circumcision as less prestigious than other, more complex medical operations that fall within their expertise, and thus they have largely performed male circumcision for pedagogical purposes only. As in the case of health officers, the practice's association with itinerant circumcisers was also another reason for doctors' reluctance concerning male circumcision. Starting in the 2000s, however, their attitude began to change, as their employers, especially private hospitals, wanted to make inroads into the circumcision market.

Private hospitals' main obstacle in attracting families for circumcision was the long-standing tradition that preserved the operation as part of the ritual. Hospitals tried to break this habit in two ways. One strategy was to add certain elements of the ritual to the operations. For instance, some hospitals began to give boys gifts and certificates as rewards for their bravery and decorated the circumcision rooms to make the hospitals warmer places for families. The other strategy was to claim that medical venues, not homes, are ideal for safe circumcision for various reasons. Hospitals were claimed to be segregated and sterilized places where operations are carried out in accordance with the principles of asepsis and antisepsis, preoperative screening (such as blood work)—missing from home-based circumcisions—is provided, and, if necessary, boys can stay overnight for further observation.

Doctors and hospitals thus sought to delegitimize health officers' credentials, expertise, and skills by raising the standards of biomedical care that health officers had introduced during the developmentalist era. This model, as we mentioned before, traced pain to tissue damage that could be prevented with professional skills, including medical knowledge and techniques. What doctors did was to broaden the range of causes of this pain and hence the appropriate expertise. For instance, they emphasized their ability to identify certain medical conditions such as hemophilia—the conditions that other practitioners would fail to notice. Some health officers and itinerant circumcisers I interviewed indeed mentioned this disorder as a cause of concern. Barber Selim, an itinerant circumciser who eventually adopted medical techniques, had encountered a few boys with hemophilia (I introduced him in chapter 1). While talking about his techniques, he said:

Allaha şükür [Thank God], I quit performing circumcision, without any accident. But I encountered five or six cases of hemophilia. Hemophilia is a disorder where the blood does not stop. I had trouble with that. Once, I cut it off, the blood did not stop. We then called a doctor. He was bruising, and the more bruised he became, the more panicked I got. It went on for a couple of days and then it stopped.

Besides pre-operation screening, doctors also emphasized that they can handle the risk of postsurgical complications better than health officers. Dr. Cengiz, a forty-five-year-old urologist, had been performing circumcision for fourteen years at a private hospital. He had not been eager to start the practice at first, though:

AUTHOR: Why didn't you want to do it at first?
CENGİZ: Pis iş [dirty job].
AUTHOR: Why did you begin, then?
CENGİZ: I did it so that circumcision would not fall into the hands of health officers and barbers.
AUTHOR: Why do you think health officers should not perform circumcision?
CENGİZ: They would have a hard time with complications. They don't have enough knowledge. Otherwise, as far as aesthetics is concerned, they perform circumcision better than doctors.
AUTHOR: What do you mean?
CENGİZ: They are obviously more experienced than us.
AUTHOR: And what kinds of complications are you talking about?
CENGİZ: For instance, allergy reactions. This happened to me once, and I could manage it. The kid had a bad allergy reaction. Health officers can't handle that. Also, as urologists, we can better diagnose and treat medical conditions, like hypospadias. You should know when you can circumcise a child and when you can't. Knowledge boosts your confidence. Knowledge is the only weapon we have in this occupation.

While Dr. Cengiz credited senior health officers for having more refined skills than doctors with limited experience in male circumcision, he added that it was only a matter of time before young doctors would catch up with health officers. And more importantly, he said, a safe operation should be more valued than a good-looking penis. Doctors can better achieve the goal of carrying out a procedure without complications than health officers, he argued, as the latter would fail to diagnose potentially life-threatening medical conditions. According to Dr. Cengiz, diagnostic skills are important, because the crucial issue in male circumcision is not only how to perform circumcision but also when and whether (or not) to perform it.[2]

As part of their efforts to delegitimize health officers, doctors also drew on the ambiguous meaning of the term *fenni sünnetçi*. Although *fenni sünnetçi* was meant to signal a clear distinction between health officers and itinerant circumcisers, the distinction grew vague, as chapter 1 showed, when itinerant circumcisers imitated health officers. Accordingly, doctors did not miss the opportunity to publicly associate health officers with itinerant circumcisers by defining *fenni sünnetçi* very broadly. My research revealed one such common description that they used: "circumciser with a bag" [çantalı sünnetçi]. Both groups of circumcisers fit into this description, since they both carried instrument bags when they went to circumcisions. Doctors often used this seemingly value-free description to refer to a circumciser of a bygone era.

Furthermore, doctors associated fenni sünnetçi with the mass circumcisions of the developmentalist era that were performed by health officers and, less often, by itinerant circumcisers. Hakan Özveri, a urologist in Acıbadem, which is the world's second-largest healthcare chain, cautioned families against mass circumcisions and fenni sünnetçi in a widely read newspaper, *Habertürk*. The news headline read: "Circumcision Shouldn't Be a Nightmare" [Sünnet Kabus Olmasın], and Özveri wrote:

> It should not be forgotten that circumcision is a surgical intervention. Thus, it should be performed by specialists in a hospital environment. Otherwise, it can cause complications and functional or cosmetic problems for the male sexual organ. Lack of concern for hygiene can increase the risk of infections. The absence of blood tests before mass circumcisions can result in missing the signs of common blood disorders and thus bleeding during operations. Besides medical problems, mass circumcisions can produce psychological problems for children. For these reasons, circumcisions should be performed only by specialists. "Fenni sünnetçi" refers to health officers or technicians who perform circumcision without medical education by using local anesthesia in medically inappropriate conditions. Today, since these techniques and approaches would lead to the problems mentioned above, they are not recommended.

Özveri's claim that health officers did not receive medical education is, of course, inaccurate. That was true of itinerant circumcisers. Nor were health officers uninformed of the relationship between male circumcision and psychology. On the contrary, as the previous chapter showed, health officers were in fact one of the pioneer groups in drawing attention to the psychological problems that male circumcision could cause. More importantly, psychological risks were among the main reasons some of them stopped participating in mass circumcision events or changed how they performed the operations (chapter 3).

They would, therefore, share Dr. Özveri's frustration over mass circumcisions. Yet, Dr. Özveri and other doctors have been successful in mobilizing the stigma attached to mass circumcisions against health officers. As a result, the fenni sünnetçi have begun to lose their prestige.

The AKP in 2015 put the final nail in the coffin of this once-highly regarded circumciser subjectivity. The government prohibited health officers' private practices, making doctors the only medical actors authorized for performing circumcision. By amending the 1928 law—the same law that once made possible the prominence of health officers in male circumcision—the government cleared the way for doctors and private hospitals to become the major players in the male circumcision market, especially in large cities. As the news headlines said: "Fenni sünnetçi is now history" (Sabah 2013).

Starting in the 2000s, then, a series of institutional, legal, and discursive transformations have supported the intrusion of private hospitals and doctors into male circumcision and the dispossession of health officers who had been serving families for decades. Moreover, the rise of the new market actors was not limited to individual circumcisions: a set of health care reforms paved the way for these actors to participate in mass circumcision events and take them over as well. Not only economic but also symbolic capital has thus become a stake in the struggles between doctors and the hospitals they work in versus health officers.

MASS CIRCUMCISIONS

In 2000, the Turkish Ministry of Health issued a new regulation on mass circumcisions. To ensure the safety of mass circumcision, the regulation demanded that sponsors receive permission from local state authorities (İl Sağlik Müdürlük) and that the operations be performed with sterilized instruments in settings maintaining the standards of asepsis and antisepsis. It also stipulated that each circumciser work with an assistant and may not perform more than eight operations per day. If sponsors hire more than one circumciser, the total number of operations per day should be limited to fifty. The total number of surgical instrument sets was required to be at least twice the total number of operations. Moreover, the code mandated that a specialist be present during the operations, ideally a urologist, or a surgeon if no urologist is available. All these changes were meant to address the much-criticized problems observed at mass circumcisions in the past: unhygienic venues and rushed operations.

The new regulation did not point to hospitals as the only venue and doctors as the main practitioners for safe mass circumcisions. However, it drastically changed the conditions under which mass circumcisions could be performed. As some health officers complained to me, a cap on the total number of operations per day and on fees for an assistant and a specialist made mass circumcisions less feasible for health officers, not to mention the fact that the new regulation officially acknowledged doctors' involvement in a supervisory capacity as essential to safe operations. The regulation thus represented a precursor to the more dramatic changes for health officers in the decades to come.

Another development that tilted the balance of power in favor of the new market actors—doctors and hospitals—was the AKP's reforms in the health care and social security system. As mentioned in chapter 3, the social security system of the developmentalist era was corporatist—rewarding only the formally employed and excluding most of the population. The benefits provided by public insurance schemes varied by occupation, and no public health care assistance scheme for the poor existed until the introduction of the Green Card in 1992—a means-tested health care program.

In 2008, the AKP transformed this system by introducing a compulsory premium-based universal health insurance scheme. Both formally employed citizens and employers were now required to pay a certain percentage of their monthly earnings into a public health insurance fund. For those who could not pay the premiums, the government extended the coverage of the Green Card. As a result of these policies, between 2003 and 2008 the coverage of premium-based health insurance grew from 59 percent to 69 percent of the total population, and the number of Green Card beneficiaries went from 2.5 million to 9.5 million (Aran and Hentschel 2012). Between 2002 and 2010, the private health expenditure of households tripled (Sönmez 2011, p. 66, as cited in Özden 2014).

In the meantime, private hospitals began to participate in mass circumcision events in collaboration with pro-Islamist municipalities in large cities. During the developmentalist era, mass circumcisions were, as shown in chapter 3, typically sponsored by nonpolitical organizations such as charitable organizations, private companies, and trade unions. In the 1990s, pro-Islamist parties began to view social assistance as an opportunity to gain, maintain, and expand political power on the level of municipalities. As part of this pro-poor political vision, these municipalities began to fund mass circumcisions in large cities, both the operations and the ritualistic aspects of the practice (such as gifts, circumcision outfits, and entertainment), and heavily publicize the events in mass media (Başaran 2021).

Starting in the 2000s, the AKP not only followed their predecessors and continued to politicize mass circumcisions but also transformed the medical side of these events into competition among hospitals. The key feature of the AKP's reforms in health care was not merely the fact that the party encouraged the growth of the private sector in health care. Rather, the reforms expanded market-based norms and metrics of success and worth into the public sector as well. The AKP has converted public hospitals into autonomous entities that are incentivized to compete against each other and other private hospitals. Moreover, the government introduced a performance system into these hospitals to increase medical professionals' productivity. All these regulations aimed to boost competition, efficiency, and consumer choice in health care services.

In the case of hospital-based mass circumcisions in large cities, public hospitals were, at least in theory, incentivized to compete against private hospitals for these operations. However, public hospitals' involvement in mass circumcisions has in practice remained limited, and the competition has mostly taken place between private hospitals. Although low-income families can bypass municipalities and have their sons circumcised free of charge at public hospitals themselves, they prefer the municipality-organized mass circumcision events in part because the municipalities provide families access to the ceremonial and celebratory components of the practice, and in large cities they therefore have private hospitals circumcise their sons.

The prize of the competition for mass circumcisions was both economic and symbolic. In 2007, the Social Security Institution (SSI), the governing authority functioning as the main consumer that buys and finances private and public health services, capped each male circumcision at an amount as low as fifty liras. Organizing mass circumcisions became an attractive opportunity for private hospitals, as they could perform procedures in large numbers and be reimbursed for each operation.

Besides the economic return on these circumcisions, symbolic profits— once similarly appropriated from itinerant circumcisers by health officers—have provided another reason for private hospitals to perform mass circumcision. By participating in these events annually, private hospitals in rural-to-urban migration neighborhoods can enhance their visibility and prestige as the carers of the poor. These hospitals have advertised on posters, pamphlets, and social media their hygienic conditions, the specialists' expertise and the state-of-the-art medical equipment and technology, and the total number of children they have circumcised over the years. Municipalities sometimes hold an auction where hospitals bid for a contract for mass circumcisions. At other times, they informally approach different hospitals in the area to get the best price for operations.

The selected private hospital would first acquire from municipalities the information of the families in need of mass circumcision assistance. A family usually applies to their municipality for this assistance with an ID, rather than going through the poverty verification process typical in other forms of social assistance. This is so because families who need the mass circumcision assistance are often beneficiaries of other social aids they receive regularly and thus are already registered in municipalities' databases. Municipalities create this database using a stringent selection process that determines whether an applicant is "deserving." The process combines formal means (official documents, rules, and procedures) with culturally and politically informed discretion on the part of municipality employees (Yoltar 2020). The hospital would then contact the "deserving" families and schedule their sons' operations. By spreading out the operations over a few days, as some health officers did in the past (chapter 3), hospitals aim to avoid rushing the operations and ensure that each boy is given due attention and proper care, both physical and psychological.

The low-income families have thus recently come under the spell of the ideology of the sovereign consumer as they have gained access to private hospitals. The appeal of private hospitals has emerged from the background of the steady defunding of public hospitals, which has resulted in long waiting lines, corruption, and low-quality service for patients with green cards. These deliberate policies set the stage for private hospitals to become a marker of prestige and status in Turkey—hence low-income families' affective investment in private hospitals for good health care and, in particular, safe circumcisions.

Do private hospitals that participate in mass circumcisions deliver what they promise? Does the appointment system work?

HOSPITAL-BASED MASS CIRCUMCISIONS

In summer 2014, I helped municipality employees working with a mass circumcision organization in Istanbul. Our job was to distribute circumcision outfits to mothers and sons, and the process was simple: we stood lined up next to each other behind the row of tables while the mothers and their sons were waiting in line on the other side, facing us. The outfits were placed in large boxes and were categorized based on age, ranging from four to eleven. We asked the mothers their sons' ages and shoe sizes, and then we handed them the outfits that would, we estimated, fit their sons. In the meantime, mothers who had been handed outfits stepped aside and quickly helped their sons try them on. When the outfits were too large or too small, mothers came back for the right sizes—a request that occasionally annoyed some municipality employees who, outside the earshot of families, used disparaging language about the mothers. They were unhappy that such requests were slowing down the process.

The distribution of outfits was followed by a celebration. On my way to the celebration, I took a taxi, as I was running late. Municipalities organize these events either before or after the operation, which may include Bosporus tours, concerts, or entertainments with clowns and games. The apex of this specific celebration, which took place before the operations, was a concert given by a nationally well-known singer. We hit heavy traffic occasioned by the celebration, and I asked the driver to drop me off two blocks away from the venue so that I could walk to the celebration. He pulled over, and as I was getting ready to get out of the car, he angrily said: "Look at these freeloaders (bedavacı)! I am sure they have more money than we do."

Both the municipality employees' and the taxi driver's language invoked the stigma typically associated with the beneficiaries of social assistance in Turkey. Since welfare benefits in Turkey are "promoted as a state benevolence rather than a citizenship right" (Yoltar 2020, p. 153), the beneficiaries are expected to feel perpetually in debt to the state. Thus, the municipality employees condemned the mothers' request for a right-sized outfit as an act of ungratefulness, and the taxi driver repeated another salient expression of this stigma that circulates widely in media. The hegemonic public discourse about the beneficiaries of social assistance always doubts the authenticity of families' claims of poverty, implying that they slyly manipulate the system. Hence, the taxi driver's assumption that the families at the mass circumcision event are impostors.

When I finally arrived at the celebration venue, the mayor was on a stage speaking in front of the families and children lying on the grass, playing, laughing, and running around. After looking around, I then started paying close attention to the mayor's speech:

> We are not leaving our families alone on their special day. We are together on this very special day. We are performing an important ceremony that carries our faith, tradition, and civilization, all these values from the past, to the future. Our children are our future. I congratulate our children and our parents. We are circumcising 250 boys this summer. Over the last fourteen years, we, as part of these annual circumcision campaigns, have circumcised thirty-eight thousand children. We have gifted circumcision outfits to our children and ensured that circumcisions have been performed in modern and hygienic conditions with state-of-the-art methods. We have completed the operations at private hospitals under the health insurance granted by our state.

Since the Istanbul municipal elections were coming soon, the mayor concluded his speech with a wish that families would support their party candidate and his promises for "our youth, children, and women." Except for this overt party propaganda, his speech was representative of mass circumcision events in contemporary Turkey: harnessing paternalistic imaginary identifications that rest upon unity and wholeness ("our," "we"), boasting the number of circumcisions as a signal of generosity, emphasizing private hospitals as a sign of good care for boys, and expressing gratitude to the state (read: AKP). Historically, however, what was new about these mass circumcisions was their venues: hospitals.

A few days later, the operations began at a private hospital. Along with other private hospitals, this hospital had been serving the migrant neighborhood since 1998. The banner draped over the hospital building said, "We are delivering circumcision services for free." Although the service is free at the point of service to families, hospitals receive fees from SSI for the operations, as described earlier. The hospital advertised the total number of mass circumcisions they had performed over the years and emphasized the hygienic conditions they provided for families. It also spread boys' circumcisions out over four days.

On the second floor of the hospital, I was waiting with families for the specialist to come and perform the operations. As time passed, the floor became crowded with families waiting for the urologist. I noticed familiar faces, as many boys were wearing the outfits we distributed. The urologist was late because he was at surgery, and one of the fathers who found out about it complained to the nurse, saying, "Why did the doctor accept another patient knowing that there are circumcisions today?" The nurse replied that there was an accident and the doctor had to perform emergency surgery. Due to the prolonged wait time, parents and their sons were getting anxious and restless.

The urologist finally arrived and rushed into the operating room while a nurse guided a boy into another room for local anesthesia and shut the door behind her. A few minutes later, the boy with the nurse started screaming and other boys who heard him burst into cries and screams, too. To calm their children, some parents shushed and reprimanded them, and others promised gifts. The closed-door seemed to function as an effective precaution to put the boy out of other boys' sight, but not to keep his voice contained. The hospital thus lacked a strategy equivalent of what Sünnetçi Yunus's clinic (chapter 4) offered: playing loud and cheerful music for each operation, to muffle, if needed, boys' screams and cries.

Once his anesthesia took effect, the crying boy was brought into the operating room by another nurse. The first nurse, who was holding the list of scheduled circumcisions, then called the next boy in the line in for local anesthesia. At the same time, the father and mother of the first boy walked into the operating room to support and calm their son, who was still scared and upset. The boy's uncle was standing by the door, straining to see around the doctor and the parents. Then the father rushed out of the room, looking pale and feeling dizzy. The uncle and a nurse held both his arms and laid him on a bed in another room. The mother also hastily walked out of the room and walked toward me: "Could you please come in to help us?" She sounded worried and panicked.

I followed the mother back into the room, where the boy on the bed was surrounded by the doctor and a male nurse. The nurse was trying to hold the boy down as the doctor was operating on him. Unfortunately, the nurse's efforts were futile, as the boy was flailing too much. The mother asked me whether I could help them to keep him stable. I joined them and grabbed one of his legs. Everyone looked away as the doctor began to cut the foreskin off. Once the operation was over, the nurse gave the boy a certificate of manhood: "[name] earned this certificate for the courage he demonstrated today. We congratulate and wish him the best of luck for the rest of his life."

The boy with tearful eyes did not seem impressed by the certificate, as he quickly handed it to his father, who was now recovered from his own minor medical problem. The boy, still crying, was ready to leave. The father asked him: "Why are you crying like a little girl?" His son remained silent. "Did you like the certificate?" the father asked, hoping to create a pleasant memory out of a rather tumultuous day. His son's response was disappointing, though: "No, I did not like it."

Soon, I would realize that the chaotic situation at the hospital was typical for the hospitals that perform mass circumcisions. The next day, I went to another hospital in another migrant neighborhood in Istanbul. On the fifth floor of the hospital, I was again waiting with families for the operations to begin. The door of the circumcision room was decorated with flowers, streamers, and a doll, and as I glanced around the room, I noticed a pile of soccer balls to be given as gifts. The urologist was late, more families were coming, and boys dressed in their circumcision outfits were getting impatient. Some were, their parents said, unusually quiet or more restless than ever, some were constantly touching their crotches, and others tightly clung to their mothers. One boy asked his mother why he had to be circumcised. "It is good for you," his mother replied. The boy did not ask why it was good for him.

The nurse announced that she would soon start administering local anesthesia according to the schedule. She asked another nurse if she knew the doctor's whereabouts. "Not sure. Maybe another surgery?" she said. As time went on, some boys became increasingly restless. A mother was dragging her son on the floor, telling him that he would not feel any pain because they were only going to measure his penis. Another boy, who saw a pen in a janitor's hand, began to cry out loud, as he mistook the pen for a circumcision instrument. "It is just a pen!" his mother replied. Then she told him to go to the circumcision room. Her son was talking to his two younger brothers, who were also going to be circumcised on the same day. The younger brothers looked much calmer. As I was watching them, the mother turned to me: "I hope his brothers will not hear him cry and get scared, too." She knew how contagious fear of male circumcision could be.

Once circumcised, boys, one after another, were walking out of the circumcision room. A mother proudly asked her son to give a soldier salute, and the son acquiesced to his mother's request with tears. "Here is your gift," his father said, handing him a toy truck that the hospital provided. "Let's go get an ice cream," he added. The boy was still crying, rubbing his eyes. Another boy came out of the circumcision room, looking much calmer than other boys. He sat next to another boy who was yet to be circumcised and mischievously told him: "They will cut off your penis."

The contrast between mass circumcisions at private hospitals in migrant neighborhoods and circumcisions at middle-class settings (clinics and private hospitals) could not be starker. Practitioners at middle-class settings acknowledge circumcision instruments to be a source of fear for boys—the fear exacerbated by the jokes that suggest excessive force—thereby seeking to mitigate the fear of circumcision by showing boys the instruments one by one. Moreover, they organized their spaces in a way to contain the contagious nature of this fear: they separated boys from each other and if necessary, isolated them, creating visible or invisible barriers between them. In doing so, they aimed to provide psychological care for boys and ensure families' satisfaction.

In contrast, the medical professionals at mass circumcisions had no time to preemptively provide comfort to boys afraid of circumcision instruments. As a result, the boy mistook a pen for a circumcision instrument, got scared, and began to cry. Moreover, it was clear that parents at the mass circumcisions were aware of the widespread discourse on trauma, as they, particularly mothers, often expressed to me their worries about the psychological effects of male circumcision on their sons. However, they were left to their own devices in handling their sons' emotions, since the crowded hospital floors did not allow for systematic and concerted fear-managing strategies to emerge. Parents tried to prevent their sons from hearing other boys' cries (sometimes by covering their ears), calm them by promising them gifts, distract them by bringing up subjects that they hoped would interest their sons (such as their favorite soccer teams), and pull them away from other crying boys. They sometimes asked the nurses (and sometimes, the researcher) to assure their sons about the safety of the operation. However, given the shortage of time and very limited space, soothing narratives about the operation could not be constructed. Nor were emotions and bodies separated, isolated, and managed efficiently.

The comparison of the two classed settings, therefore, demonstrates strikingly opposite temporal and spatial organizations of male circumcision. On the one hand, space at the middle-class settings expands, differentiates, and multiplies via visible and invisible walls, and time unfolds in a linear manner, with a clear beginning and an end. No interruption of the well-orchestrated and well-planned series of acts and events is tolerated. At the hospital-based mass circumcisions, on the other hand, the space shrinks, and bodies are trapped, and time is simultaneously experienced as too fast and too slow: circumcisions are at once delayed and rushed due to the limited time to finish all scheduled operations, while every single stage of the operation becomes too demanding, repetitive, and exhausting. When boys flail too much, health professionals start over. Parents try to calm their sons repeatedly. Time does not feel to be moving. While the strategies of middle-class circumcision venues are proactive, systematic, and collective, their counterparts at mass circumcisions are reactive, thereby turning into forced improvisations and makeshift solutions—an outcome of a combination of too much fear and too limited resources.

Health professionals at mass circumcisions are influenced by the psychological discourse of trauma and yet perform the operations under conditions unsuitable for providing what they consider proper medical care—especially psychological care. How do health professionals cope with the conflict between their ethical values about care and what the immediate situation demanded?

THE DECEITFUL CHILD AND PARENT-BLAMING

I observed another mass circumcision, performed by Dr. Tekin, a fifty-five-year-old urologist at a private hospital in Istanbul. The hospital had been serving the residents of the migrant neighborhood for fifteen years and had been performing mass circumcisions for five years. As always, I was chatting with families and waiting for the operations to begin. For this specific mass circumcision event, the municipality had organized the celebration before the operations, and the boys at the hospital were wearing their casual outfits. That said, the hospital had still decorated the operating room with gifts, and certificates were ready for the boys.

Dr. Tekin was two hours late for the first operation, and the floor was already crammed with boys and their families. At one point, the floor's capacity was exceeded, and one of the nurses began to ask the arriving families to wait outside the hospital. Another nurse announced that the operations would begin soon and called in the first boy for local anesthesia. Coincidentally, I was talking to the same boy's parents, who had invited me to the operation. After the anesthesia, the nurse took the boy, Ferhat, to the operating room. Ferhat's parents and I were standing by the operating bed as they tried to comfort their son, who looked very nervous and was shaking. As Dr. Tekin began to work on the foreskin, Ferhat started crying out, "It hurts! It hurts!" Dr. Tekin, frustrated over his reaction, said, "Look, I am not even doing anything. I am now only pressing it [scalpel blade] against your foreskin. That's it." As Dr. Tekin kept pressing it, the boy continued saying that it hurt. The doctor got very upset, responding dismissively, "No, it does not. You are making it up!" He looked at me and the parents and said, "It is just fear." Then, he scolded the parents, "This is your fault, you know, right? I am sure you have family problems, and your boy is influenced by them. Or did you scare him before you came here?"

Dr. Tekin's dialogue with me and the parents invoked two main tropes: the Deceitful Child and Bad Parents. When Dr. Tekin pressed the tip of the blade against Ferhat's penis, Ferhat gave a very common reaction to the sensation of cold he felt. Health professionals are widely familiar with this reaction: as we saw in the previous chapter, circumcisers typically tell boys before the operation that they should expect this sensation. By doing so, they seek to strike off an item from the list of what might shock boys. However, Dr. Tekin did not prepare Ferhat for what would happen during the operation, scolded him for lying about his pain, and dismissed his pain by calling it "just" a fear.

Dr. Tekin's reaction was undoubtedly harsh, but not an anomaly. Other health professionals I observed at mass circumcisions also often invoked the figure of the Deceitful Child: a child who exaggerates his pain and manipulates the circumciser and his family. As another doctor said:

> They [children] skillfully manipulate their parents. This is especially true for boys with divorced parents. I feel really bad for those kids. They sense that their parents are extra sensitive toward them because of, you know, the separation, and they think that they can get their way by crying.

While the trauma-based model of harm grants a distinct ontological status and moral legitimacy to emotions and calls for their management for the sake of boys' well-being, biological reductionism allows health professionals to question the certainty of others' pain and suffering as well as refute the veracity of, and trivialize, their reports: if no underlying physiological causes of pain can be detected, then the pain does not exist. As long as a health professional uses local anesthesia, , like Dr. Tekin did, then the pain expressed by boys can be written off as unreal or illegitimate: "It is just fear," or "You are not in pain, you are making it up."

The Deceitful Child, in other words, emerges as a figure onto which health professionals displace the anxiety regarding care, harm, and responsibility that also shapes their interactions with families and the care they provide. It serves as an ideological and affective defense against what would otherwise unsettle health professionals—a defense through which they regress to biomedical reductionism. Health professionals at mass circumcisions believe that they are providing proper biomedical care, as proven by all physical markers of pain and suffering, such as lack of bleeding. Sure, their reductionism suggests, boys still express pain, but expressions are a matter of language and mind and are therefore subject to deception and self-deception. Such expressions are not reliable. The figure of the Deceitful Child thus evokes the mind-body dualism that locates the pain either in the mind or the body: when it is the former, as in the case of fear, it can then legitimately be ignored.

However, given the widespread influence of the trauma-based model in male circumcision over the last decades, health professionals cannot always simply dismiss boys' expressions of pain and suffering as unreal or illegitimate. The model has become so ingrained into how they assess the safety of circumcisions that boys' emotional discomfort and outbursts, taken as disturbing signs of failure, continue to put emotional pressure on health professionals. Here, another ideological figure comes into the picture—a figure that does not discredit boys' suffering but still allows health professionals to project the responsibility of this suffering onto others: the Bad Parents.

On a different occasion, I was chatting with families at another private hospital that carried out mass circumcisions via an appointment system. Again, the urologist who was going to perform the operations was late, and the floor became overcrowded very quickly. Some boys were standing and restless, others were quiet. A mother to whom I talked earlier turned to me and her relatives and said, "He [her son] did not sleep all night. He was very excited. In the morning, he insisted that his sister should come too." His son, Selim, indeed looked calmer than other boys. Then, we heard another boy who was getting local anesthesia start crying while his parents were trying to calm him down. Selim, perplexed by what was happening, asked, "What are these noises, mom?" His mom said it was nothing. As the noises became louder, Selim lost his calmness and eagerness. He also broke into tears and refused to be circumcised.

The urologist finally arrived. Selim's father grabbed him and took him to a circumcision room as Selim was trying to free himself from his father's grasp. Selim's uncles also went into the room. Selim's mother anxiously covered her mouth and said to her husband, "I can't look at it." She decided to stand outside the circumcision room and, seeing another boy walking out of another circumcision room, congratulated him. Selim was lying on the bed, surrounded by nurses, the urologist, his father, and his uncles. Everyone was trying to hold Selim down so that the urologist could comfortably and safely circumcise him. Selim was screaming for his mother to come in as well. His mother could not move an inch, as she felt weighed down. One of the uncles came out, saying, "This is like a sacrificial lamb [kurbanlık koyun]! Three people are holding him!" He then went back in, and a couple of minutes later, the boy's father walked out hastily. "I can't really take this," he said. "He is screaming." He never went back inside. Once the operation was over, the urologist rushed out of the room to get ready for the next operation. The nurse was holding Selim's hand when all of them came out of the room. Selim wiped his tears off with his sleeves while the nurse was instructing his mother about postoperative care: no shower for twenty-four hours, apply antibiotic ointment, and painkillers may be used in case he feels pain.

The uncle's words ("this is like a sacrificial lamb") comparing his nephew's circumcision to animal sacrifice exposed a hidden continuity between mass circumcisions in the past and the present. As shown in chapter 3, various actors such as religious leaders and health authorities have condemned the ways animals are slaughtered as part of Eid al-Adha in large cities, pointing out the unhygienic venues and animals' unnecessary suffering in the hands of incompetent butchers. Around the same time, health professionals began to compare mass circumcisions organized in nonmedical settings to animal sacrifice as a way to dramatize the problems observed at mass circumcisions. In both cases, one of the targets of criticism was migrant families (the other one was health officers), who were seen as failing the "litmus test" of modern citizenship and were considered responsible for avoidable suffering in both animals and children. Selim's uncle, thus, inadvertently invoked the very stigma that had been hovering over migrant families like his for decades. His words also revealed the failure of hospital-based mass circumcisions to change the organization of these operations: overcrowded nonmedical settings were merely replaced with overcrowded hospital floors.

On that day, Selim and the other boys had been circumcised by Dr. Mehmet, a forty-five-year-old doctor. Dr. Mehmet had been performing circumcision, both mass and individual, for fifteen or sixteen years, first as an assistant and then as a general surgeon. I talked to him right after he completed all the circumcisions scheduled for the day. He was exhausted and very bitter about mass circumcisions:

MEHMET: Let me make something clear first. This is a special occasion. Normally, I perform two or three circumcisions per week. Now we perform thirty or forty circumcisions per day. Municipalities organize these circumcisions. This is partly about benevolence but also partly about marketing. If you are asking for my opinion as a doctor: I do not approve of it. But you know, we have to perform these circumcisions, because the hospitals are requiring us to. Circumcision is a medical operation, and it should be taken seriously. Of course, we sterilize our instruments one by one and do our best to prevent contamination. But in these situations, I can't understand children's psychology. Or even if I understand them, I can't pay attention to them. But under normal circumstances, I first talk to children, and if I feel like they are not ready for circumcision psychologically, I recommend general anesthesia. Educated families ask me about the operation. They read about circumcision on the internet, and they actually talk to their sons and inform them about the operation. If they are old enough, children understand what their families say to them.

AUTHOR: But this is not the case in mass circumcisions, I guess?

MEHMET: No. Since they do not pay anything for these circumcisions, they do not care about whether anything would happen to their sons, like psychological trauma.

Dr. Mehmet emphasized the dual aspects of mass circumcisions: benevolence and marketing. By "marketing," he was referring to both political and economic motivations, as political parties and private hospitals have instrumentalized mass circumcisions for electoral success and economic and symbolic gains. Dr. Mehmet was against mass circumcisions but without any discretionary power over how, let alone whether, to organize and perform them. In his view, middle-class families are educated enough to make informed decisions about circumcision and to know how to communicate with their sons about the operation.

Yet, the migrant families at mass circumcisions, he suggested, are unconcerned about their sons' well-being because the operations are free (although the above vignettes illustrating families' worries regarding their sons' emotions show that his assumption was groundless). Thus, Mehmet held the families, rather than the hospitals, responsible for the lack of psychological care at mass circumcisions—a problem that unsettled his ethical values about care and harm and his status as a medical professional. Another urologist, Dr. Basri, echoed Mehmet's sentiments.

Dr. Basri, born in 1972, had been working at the same private hospital as a general surgeon for seven years and had been performing circumcision for ten years. He and other doctors usually performed three or four hundred circumcisions each year during the summer and a few neonatal circumcisions throughout the rest of the year. He had to have his son circumcised at the age of one due to an infection, but he would otherwise, he said, have waited until an age when the boy could remember his circumcision. "Would you ever consider not having him circumcised at all if you had another son?" I asked him. "No," he said. He would, he added, be worried that his son would face discrimination later in his life.

Dr. Basri himself was circumcised at his village by an itinerant circumciser, without local anesthesia. He remembered crying after the operation, but he has no memory of feeling pain. "My recovery was long, though," he said. "Now, the recovery is much shorter, since we are using stitches," he added. Unlike some other doctors, he prefers local anesthesia over general anesthesia, since the latter, he thinks, is too risky for young children. I asked him about mass circumcisions as well:

AUTHOR: How are mass circumcisions different from other circumcisions?
BASRI: They are different both technically and in terms of communication.
AUTHOR: Why technically?
BASRI: You must be faster. It is the same system, but, for instance, we do fewer stitches because we must do it quickly. We have less time at these circumcisions. The more stitches, the faster the healing becomes. There might also be some issues regarding sterilization, but not many.
AUTHOR: And you always circumcise them under local anesthesia?
BASRI: Yes, of course. The equipment is the same. The problem is mostly communication.
AUTHOR: What about it?
BASRI: We interact with kids much less. Normally, we talk to kids about the operation. We tell them the steps of the operation. We can't really do that here, because we need to be fast. Families also do not prepare their kids. On the morning of the day when circumcision will happen, they scare their sons. They do not see that they are dealing with a kid. And when kids get scared, they say, "Son, why are you scared?" They don't care. They think that it is a simple operation. This is a serious operation.

Dr. Basri seemed confident about the biomedical care he was providing at mass circumcision, though he noted a need for an improvement on that front as well. His major concern was psychological. Boys at the two types of circumcisions, individual and mass, share similarly anxious thoughts about circumcision instruments and male circumcision in general. However, at mass circumcisions Dr. Basri did not have enough time to talk to boys, answer their questions, and clear the misconceptions they might have regarding the instruments and the operation in general.

With the incorporation of the trauma-based model into male circumcision, the metrics of success and failure for health professionals changed: the elimination of not only physical pain, as was the case in biomedicalization, but also emotional discomfort, fear, and anxiety. Ideally, health professionals and families would work in concert to protect boys' well-being and prevent their fear from condensing into trauma. Yet, in dire situations like mass circumcisions where operations are haphazardly performed, cooperation can give way to conflict, if not outright hostility, between the two actors—especially if one party (in this case, health professionals) tends to have ideological baggage about the other party. Medical professionals thus expressed frustration about hospitalized mass circumcisions where, compared to individual circumcisions, they felt that they could not provide enough psychological care and often, implicitly or explicitly, either denied boys' suffering or blamed families for it.

Health professionals' ideological baggage about families is based on the category of the "deserving" poor. As the bureaucratically governed social assistance programs have become the new welfare norm during the neoliberal period in Turkey, poverty has become a fact to be managed rather than eradicated. The AKP has normalized the assumption of scarce resources, thereby rendering a significant portion of the population—especially urban migrants—morally suspect: a family is not poor until they prove otherwise. The authenticity of the migrants' claims of poverty and their moral integrity has thus come under harsh scrutiny, not only by state officials but also by the public in general. The beneficiaries of social assistance have come to be seen as ignorant, manipulative, and self-interested freeloaders, and finally, in the case of male circumcision, as irresponsible parents who would jeopardize their sons' health by having them circumcised at mass circumcision events.

BEYOND IDEOLOGY

Medical sociologists and anthropologists have shown that when working under resource-poor conditions, medical professionals (for instance, doctors and nurses), who otherwise acknowledge the importance of the biopsychosocial model, often resort, consciously or nonconsciously, to the biomedical reductionism that typically goes hand in hand with the stigma around certain groups. This is especially the case when they navigate moral and professional challenges, feel pressured to justify their choices of certain treatments and not others, or assess who deserves urgent care and who does not (Bridges 2011; Brodwin 2013; Buchbinder 2015; Morande 2019; Reich 2014; Timmermans 1998; Ware 1992). They may see the "undesirables"—for instance, the poor, addicts, the homeless, the elderly, and women with chronic fatigue syndrome—as a burden on the society, blaming them for draining its resources (time and money), which, they believe, could otherwise be used more efficiently for others. Poor women of color can be considered as "unruly bodies" (Bridges 2011) in need of excessive medicalization and pathologizing surveillance, while the nonpoor can utilize more holistic approaches to care. Or, health professionals can tell those with chronic pain that it is all in their head, dismissing the legitimacy of their suffering as undetected by physiological markers (Buchbinder 2015).

Similarly, this chapter draws attention to a class setting where health professionals, working with limited resources (especially time), fail to provide what they consider proper care for boys. In contrast to the middle-class settings where health professionals are demanded to deliver more than what is possible, health professionals at mass circumcisions deliver less than what is possible. As in the case of the developmentalist era, the bodies of the poor have again become anonymous in settings where individualized attention to boys remains an unfulfilled promise. The health professionals at these settings thus find themselves in moral agony, as they cannot reconcile their ethical values concerning medical care—particularly psychological care—with their working conditions. To manage this agony, they tend to cast boys and their families as moral suspects by combining the widespread stigma about migrant families with a reductionist biomedical model of care and pain.

Our case thus demonstrates that the nature of the medical model—biomedical or biopsychosocial—applied in a given setting is not merely a question of medical education or intention on the part of health professionals; rather, it depends on available resources, power relations, and ideologies within that setting. More specifically, the Deceitful Child and Bad Parents both serve as interpretive grids and affective anchors whereby health professionals extract themselves from the deadlock they face and continue ambivalently to bind themselves to their professional values and prestige: they identify with the psychologist-by-proxy only by distancing themselves from it as they seek to absolve themselves of any responsibility for boys' suffering. In doing so, they can confront the pressure (read: guilt) stemming from performing circumcisions under adverse conditions. These figures are ideological in the sense that they conceal, and divert attention from, the structural roots of the problems observed at mass circumcisions: the concentration of male circumcision demands in the hands of fewer and fewer competing medical actors. Thus, rather than resorting to these well-worn ideological figures, health professionals could have provided a different account for why they cannot achieve their goals at mass circumcisions.

Dr. Mehmet indeed offered a glimpse of such an account when he emphasized the relationship between mass circumcisions and marketing. He implied a causal link between overcrowded hospitals and political and economic competition. But we can ponder these issues further. The rise of private hospitals, as mentioned earlier, has been a key development in recent decades in Turkey and part of a broader and wide-ranging transformation of the health care system under the AKP. One of the outcomes of the AKP reforms in health care has been that health professionals at hospitals have increasingly found themselves in precarious employment and working conditions as these hospitals have introduced a stricter disciplinary regime to optimize efficiency and productivity. This has meant longer and more flexible working hours for health professionals and a decrease in the allocated time for each patient (Agartan 2015).

The shortage of time in health care has been a chronic problem in Turkey, as the lack of a strong primary care network and the sudden spike in access to hospitals has put a lot of pressure on health professionals—especially those who serve low-income neighborhoods. Specialists have begun to see patients with minor problems that otherwise would normally be handled by primary caregivers. Moreover, health professionals have also been encouraged to lean toward performing more surgeries than in the past. As a result, although the number of providers has grown, so have their patient loads. Between 2002 and 2019, the total number of working physicians increased by 75 percent. However, in the same period, the average patient started to make considerably more frequent visits to various medical providers and facilities. In 2002, the average patient visited their doctor around three times per year, but by 2019, the numbers of annual visits had grown to nine or ten. Similarly, people now go to public hospitals six times per year instead of twice, and private hospital visits per capita have grown from 0.1 to 0.9. During these years, the annual number of surgical operations increased by almost 600 percent (Health Statistics Yearbook 2019). All of these statistics show a significant increase in health professionals' workload.

In the case of mass circumcisions, the exclusion of health officers from male circumcision and the competition between hospitals for economic and symbolic capital have typically moved these circumcisions to one or two hospitals in a neighborhood, which are already overwhelmed by other health care demands. This monopolization explains why all the urologists in the above vignettes were behind schedule and therefore rushed the operations. Like health officers during the developmentalist era, these doctors had to move from one boy to another very quickly. But unlike the mass circumcisions in the past, the shortage of time in mass circumcisions now risks, in the eyes of health professionals, not only physical but also psychological harm. And rather than blaming boys who supposedly manipulate adults and families who supposedly have no regard for the safety of their sons, critical scrutiny could be directed at the market-oriented policies, privatization, and commodification leading to the persistent infrastructural deficiencies of mass circumcisions.

Today, circumcision operations (mass or individual) in Turkey typically take place at hospitals and are separated from celebrations. Medical professionals such as urologists, with the assistance of a medical team, perform the operations under either local or general anesthesia, depending on boys' ages and their families' preferences. Moving even further to minimize pain or trauma, middle-class parents in large cities increasingly prefer neonatal circumcisions. Health officers' private practices have, like the recent ban on health officers intended, largely disappeared, though some perform circumcision at hospitals in small cities and towns. Consequently, the revenue from male circumcision has been transferred from health officers to hospitals—especially private hospitals in large cities. Municipalities, benevolent individuals, and NGOs continue to sponsor mass circumcision events for low-income families at hospitals, while other families organize their own celebrations with extended families and neighbors.

THE ETHICS AND POLITICS
OF MALE CIRCUMCISION

This book operationalizes a psychoanalytically informed sociological notion of ambivalence to make sense of the contradictions of the changing subjectivity of circumcisers in Turkey. It suggests that dominant sociological approaches to subjectivity fail to attend to the paradoxical nature of subjectivity, which integrates what it disavows. In medical sociology, the basic psychoanalytical notion of the self-sabotaging subject can, I claim, help us theorize the kinds of transformations that subjects must go through to fashion themselves as the agents of medicalization. In doing so, I avoid taking for granted circumcisers' desire for medicalization and demonstrate that their relationship with the medicalization process is far from straightforward. Instead, circumcisers have been a stake, as as much an agent, of medicalization.

In each period of medicalization, identification with the position of Sünnetçi has had the lurking potential of transgressing norms, undermining professional values, and violating prescriptions by coming across as too greedy, being mistaken for others, losing (self-)respect, and harming boys—all of which exert pressure on nerves, self-images, and relationships with others. And I argue that, through fantasies such as "Traditional Authority" (chapter 1), "Fenni Sünnetçi" (chapter 2), "Carers of the Poor" (chapter 3), the "Strategy of Splitting" (chapter 4), and the "Deceitful Child" and "Bad Parents" (chapter 5), circumcisers, discursively and organizationally, have confronted this pressure. Put differently, circumcisers have, paradoxically, identified themselves with historically produced subject positions such as "scientific circumciser," "caring circumciser," and "benevolent circumciser" by distancing themselves from them. Ambivalences have been key to their subjectivities.

Rather than reiterating all the points made in the preceding chapters in further detail, what follows will discuss the sociological insights that can be gleaned from the Turkish circumcision case for the ongoing circumcision debate internationally. Male circumcision has recently become a matter of ethical and political debate among health professionals, politicians, NGOs, lawmakers, and academics all around the world. My goal is to reflect on the significance of circumcisers' ambivalent attachments to medicalization in Turkey for this debate, as these attachments are shaped around *ethics of care* and *status*. I argue that circumcisers' ambivalences indicate that economic policies, health inequalities, and ideologies should be part of the circumcision debate if we want to broaden our ethical and political horizon concerning male circumcision in Turkey and elsewhere.

THE CIRCUMCISION DEBATE

Male circumcision has sparked controversies in recent decades in various countries, albeit much less so in Turkey. In Europe, the German regional court in Cologne in 2012 decided to prohibit the circumcision of minors. The court reasoned that removing healthy tissue from an infant is, in the absence of any net health benefit, unethical and a violation of their human rights. In a similar vein, in 2018 Iceland's Progressive Party proposed a bill to prohibit male circumcision, claiming that the practice harmed the bodily integrity of young boys and was thus incompatible with the United Nations Convention on the Rights of the Child. The ban on male circumcision never took effect in either country but set off a debate over the legitimacy of male circumcision: is nontherapeutic male circumcision morally permissible?

On the humanitarian and public health front, the United Nations Joint Programme on HIV/AIDS (UNAIDS) and the World Health Organization (WHO) in 2007 recommended male circumcision to reduce the risk of acquiring HIV infection. As part of a campaign between 2008 and 2018, 23 million boys and men in eastern and southern Africa underwent what the WHO calls "voluntary medical male circumcision" (VMMC) (Dickson et al. 2011). Since then, this campaign has been criticized on scientific, ethical, political, and public health grounds for encouraging unprotected sex, exaggerating the benefits of the operation, and making behavioristic assumptions about HIV and overlooking its structural causes (Berer 2007; Drash 2019; Garenne et al. 2013).

In Muslim countries such as Turkey and Egypt, the anticircumcision camp emphasizes the nonobligatory status of male circumcision in Islam and even goes so far as to define it as a crime against humanity and religion (el-Sharkawy 2019). In the US, the group Intact America opposes coerced genital cutting on persons of any age or gender, defining it as psychically and psychologically harmful, and runs campaigns and organizes protests to raise awareness about the issue.[1] They argue that the evidence for its health benefits is weak and, more importantly, inconsequential, as basic hygiene routines (for instance, cleaning one's foreskin regularly) can produce the same health benefits (such as reduced risk of cancer) that male circumcision is said to produce, but without the physical and psychological burden.

While international institutions have rightly fought female genital mutilation, the anticircumcision camp argues, they have been long overdue in
putting an end to what the "intactivists" (as some refer to themselves) call "male
child genital cutting." Just as the partial or total removal of external female
genitalia is a cruel practice diminishing girls' autonomy over their bodies, they
emphasize, so is the partial or total removal of the foreskin that is carried out
without boys' consent and against their best interests.

These polarized and moralized public disputes over male circumcision
often frame male circumcision via supposedly self-evident lenses such as
"rights," "culture," "public health," and "risk"—the same lenses that inform
much of the academic writings on the topic as well. For instance, following
the German court decision, the *Journal of Medical Ethics* published a series of
articles expressing polarized views on the matter. In his piece, Joseph Mazor
(2013) argues against the court decision as justified on the grounds of the
child's interests, self-determination, and right to bodily integrity. In the case of
religiously motivated circumcisions where the practice is rooted in communal
ties, Mazor claims, one can safely assume that the child is likely to choose to
become circumcised as an adult member of the community in the future. It
is thus in the child's interest, so his reasoning goes, to have boys circumcised
as infants to reduce health risks and the discomfort they would experience if
they were to undergo the procedure as adults.

Mazor also contests the argument that male circumcision violates children's right to bodily integrity by pointing out that parents often make decisions about their children's health and appearance that can be construed
as violating the same right. Consider, he says, children born with cleft lips,
a minor problem that does not warrant an operation on the lips for purely
medical reasons. However, parents who are concerned about their children
being mocked at school sometimes have their children's lips fixed. The same
rationale, the author claims, can also be used in the case of male circumcision,
since uncircumcised boys can suffer peer pressure in a community where male
circumcision is a norm.

Other philosophers, such as Matthew Thomas Johnson (2013) and Brian D.
Earp (2013), disagree with Mazor, arguing that a proper secular and liberal
approach should take a neutral stance regarding religious and cultural values,
and thus it is unfair to advocate the eradication of female genital cutting
while exempting male genital cutting from criticism. Both practices, they say,
diminish children's autonomy, subject them to the will of their communities,
and violate children's rights. Regardless of their ethical stance, scholars of
both camps tend to agree that a blanket criminalization of male circumcision
would be unhelpful and harmful to boys, since families who have a strong

commitment to the tradition would then have their sons circumcised by un-qualified practitioners under unhygienic conditions.

The academic and public controversy over male circumcision reveals tensions unique to the liberal political thinking around rights and freedom, which attempts to balance children's rights to self-determination and bodily integrity, and their autonomy from families and communities, with parents' religious freedom and rights. The opposing positions show that these much-cherished liberal values are not static but open to interpretation and do not readily translate to policies and moral consensus. Ethical concerns about harm, care, and human flourishing imbue the circumcision debate with different and sometimes conflicting assumptions about "the good life."

ORDINARY ETHICS

A standard social scientific contribution to the debate would entail breaking away from the abstract and formal principles and values (for instance, autonomy) that shape the circumcision debate and calling for attention to actors' moral reflections on immediate and practical activities. Scholars argue that rather than resorting to hypothetical scenarios, as is often seen in bioethics, or reified abstractions such as human rights, we should examine the "ordinary ethics" buried in real-life settings—a mundane form of ethics that is "relatively tacit, grounded in agreement rather than the rule, in practice rather than knowledge or belief, and happening without calling undue attention to itself" (Lambek 2010, p. 2). Ordinary ethics can, it is claimed, give us a better sense of what people value and see as urgent in their everyday lives.

In medicine, the ordinary ethics perspective can indeed help generate important sociological insights about organizations. Medical sociologists and anthropologists point out that ethics in medicine is dominated by a highly professionalized branch of ethics, namely bioethics (Chambliss 1996; Kaufman 1997; Kleinman 2006). Much of bioethics, they point out, assumes the centrality of autonomous decision-makers engaging in hypothetical scenarios that have little value for dealing with routine yet life-changing problems. Bioethics carries the traces of professional hierarchies, as it is often written by the powerful: for instance, doctors. It inevitably omits the vantage point of the less powerful, such as nurses, who engage in practical ethical dilemmas and uncertainties daily. More importantly, they often do so without having any decision-making power over the problems they face. Paying attention to the low-ranked members of organizations thus can help us broaden the range of ethical questions we can ask and of organizational problems we can identify and change.

Notwithstanding its merits, the ordinary ethics approach, as anthropologist Paul Brodwin (2013) argues, might draw an overly neat distinction between the abstract and the concrete, the universal and the local, the explicit and the tacit, and the formal and the informal. Analyzing the ethical dilemmas of frontline mental health staff serving the most destitute, Brodwin shows how clinical work is shaped by the categories and values of bioethics, such as patient autonomy. In reflecting on their work experiences and their rather difficult decisions about patients, the staff members invoke these moral categories and values. As a result, bioethics becomes written into the fabric of the local moral worlds at the clinics rather than remaining, as the ordinary ethics approach might imply, as experience-distant abstract instructions.

With this caveat in mind, throughout the book I have shown that the ordinary ethics approach can help shed new light on the male circumcision debate. Ethics is contextually situated and historically produced, as the standards of proper circumcision have changed over time. Moreover, moral values concerning care have manifested themselves as much in explicit statements, laws, and codes as in circumcisers' visceral reactions, dilemmas, and struggles, all of which are enmeshed with economic interests and hierarchies of power and prestige. While the circumcision debate engages in abstract philosophical speculation that limits the ethical and political horizon regarding male circumcision to "for" or "against" options, the close analysis of how circumcisers have encountered the pressure of the structure of inequalities and reflected on practical matters concerning care—on what is right and wrong and the obligatory and the forbidden—can, I suggest, bring forth new questions and elaborations about the ethics and politics of male circumcision.

ETHICS AND MALE CIRCUMCISION IN TURKEY

Throughout the history of the medicalization of male circumcision in Turkey, circumcisers' moral concerns regarding medical care have arisen from local and diverse contexts shaped by changing health care laws and policies, new scientific discourses, and enduring class-based inequalities. Chapter 2 discussed the ruling elites' conflicting views over the fate of male circumcision as a religious practice in the early republican period: Should the new modern state that takes European civilization as a model endorse a "barbaric" practice? How can the goal of population health be achieved if male circumcision puts children's bodily integrity at risk? These questions culminated in a law in 1928 that codified moral concerns about care, harm, and health within the paradigm of modern medicine—the law that set the stage for health professionals, starting in the 1960s, to disseminate via mass media the new medicalized circumcision ethos focusing on pain.

In the post–World II era, the ethos inscribed into the 1928 law shaped health officers' conflicts in their everyday lives. Medical professionals during the developmentalist era were, as shown in chapters 2 and 3, motivated partly to gain power and prestige and partly to provide better care for boys than itinerant circumcisers did. The social security system of the time excluded the majority of the society, creating the conditions for mass circumcisions to become a matter of competition among health officers who wanted to make a name in their communities. Yet, health officers at these operations could not deliver the kind of care they deemed ideal for boys: they rushed the operations, rarely sterilized the instruments, and never provided follow-up care.

Starting in the 2000s, as shown in chapter 4, psychologists in Turkey started expressing their opinions in mass media on the potential psychological effects of male circumcision on boys. They introduced a new trauma-based language and criticized fear-inducing habits around male circumcision within society, without calling for an end to the practice. In dialogue with this new discourse and its implicit moral imperatives, circumcisers recalibrated their ethical views about what constituted harm and care for boys in male circumcision and developed new techniques and practices to sustain boys' psychological well-being. Around the same time, doctors (as the new faces of medical authority) and private hospitals (as the new circumcision venues) began to replace health officers and homes, respectively.

The incorporation of psychological care into neoliberal consumerism has generated two main class-based outcomes for medical professionals and families. The middle-class settings demand that health professionals exercise constant vigilance over unpleasant and fear-inducing interactions, images, sounds, and words. Providing psychological care is now enmeshed with sustaining consumer satisfaction and comfort. On the rare occasions I observed when a crisis, such as an emotional outburst, occurred, health professionals' visceral reactions were hard to miss. They panicked when a boy was about to cry and aimed to either prevent it or hide it from sight, as families could take this as a sign of failure.

At hospital-based mass circumcisions, as shown in chapter 5, the same risk of failure has lost its urgent character, and health professionals' panic concerning mistakes has given way to a sense of resignation, a bitter acceptance of the ordinariness of what would otherwise be dramatized as a crisis at a middle-class venue. The AKP introduced market mechanisms into the health care system to boost competition and efficiency while channeling circumcisions, including mass circumcisions, toward hospitals. On the one hand, low-income families, once relegated to informal security mechanisms during the developmentalist era, finally became integrated into the formal social security system during the neoliberal era. On the other hand, as health officers gradually discontinued their private practices and were eventually banned from practice, the market-oriented model of health care led to the concentration of male circumcisions in the hands of even fewer competing actors, namely hospitals (especially private hospitals in large cities)—a process that, paradoxically, has culminated in reproducing the very problem that the hospital system of circumcisions was meant to solve: overcrowded circumcision venues. At this time, hospital floors, rather than nonmedical settings of the developmentalist era, are becoming packed with families. Now, instead of health officers, doctors find themselves grappling with the tension between their collective medical ethos—now defined by both biomedical and psychological models of care—and their working conditions. Their daily hospital practices are constantly troubled by disruptions and failures.

Furthermore, I have shown that class inequalities have manifested themselves in not only the different spatial and temporal configurations of circumcision events but also in the implicit judgments over who deserves immediate attention and who does not. In attempting to reorganize the society according to market mechanisms, the neoliberal social, economic, cultural, and political transformation has taken poverty as a natural fact to be managed, assumed the resources to be scarce, and infused social assistance with bias and prejudice. In the developmentalist era, rural-to-urban migrants were widely seen as the "disadvantaged Other" (Erman 2001) and poverty as an outcome of economic inequalities. However, the dominant political discourses and cultural representations over the last three decades have equated being poor with moral failure and labeled the migrants as "the undeserving Others" (Erman 2001). This ideological transformation accounts for health professionals' response to their ethical conflicts around care at hospital-based mass circumcisions: doctors I observed invoked the widespread notion of the poor as sly and manipulative subjects, blaming families for the low quality of medical care the doctors provided.

I have demonstrated that circumcisers' ambivalences have shaped how they have viewed themselves with respect to inequalities embedded within relations of dispossession, exclusion, inclusion, and competition. They have made affective investments in certain practices, strategies, interactions, and discourses in order to gain, maintain, or recover status, and each transformation of subjectivity has represented a distinct configuration of ambivalences unique to different historical contexts. And these ambivalences at times have become a basis of positive social change as well. For instance, as we saw in chapter 3, some health officers began to reorganize mass circumcision in the 1980s and 1990s to redress the problem of the low-quality care they were providing to low-income families. In doing so, they gave a different response to the pressure of guilt than have other health officers, such as those who decided to quit performing mass operations altogether.

Focusing on circumcisers' moral ambivalences suggests that economic policies, health inequalities, and ideologies should be part of the circumcision debate, as it can help us envision a new set of political interventions in male circumcision. On the one hand, the pro-circumcision camp defends male circumcision as a legitimate practice but fails to take into account the stratified nature of the society, assuming that actors (practitioners and families) experience male circumcision across social settings in a uniform manner. On the other hand, the advocates of the anti-circumcision camp do not see male circumcision as a morally permissible practice but acknowledge that, as mentioned earlier, families would not give up on their long-standing tradition overnight. Hence, a blanket ban would be counterproductive. Accordingly, some have recommended reforms of harm reduction such as mandatory administration of anesthesia to reduce risk, pain, and suffering in male circumcision.

However, the case of male circumcision in Turkey has demonstrated that such harm reduction policies would still fall short of generating the intended outcomes unless the existing health inequalities are addressed. Both the state-centered and market-oriented health care models in Turkey have excluded a considerable segment of practitioners and deprived low-income families of what counts as good quality medical care—inequalities prevalent in other circumcision-practicing countries as well. Male circumcision per se has not typically arisen as an ethical problem among families and practitioners. When I asked my interviewees for their thoughts about the common critiques of male circumcision, they dismissed the critiques and justified the practice on the grounds of religion, custom, and health. The pressing issue for them was to carry out the operations without causing physical and psychological harm to boys. They reflected on how their circumstances are shaped by inequalities via the notion of safe circumcision, rather than in terms of the liberal language of autonomy and freedom—language that has dominated the larger circumcision debate.

Given that male circumcision now takes place in medical settings, moral issues around the practice can't be separated from broader infrastructural problems unique to the health care system: insufficient resources, overworked health professionals, and overcrowded medical venues. Accordingly, we can claim that policies that would address the persisting unequal distribution of health care services including medicalized male circumcision, such as the expansion of those eligible to perform circumcision and the range of circumcision venues, would benefit not only low-income boys but also those health professionals who find themselves in poor working conditions. Similarly, changing the cultural environment around care to cultivate a capacity for living with medical uncertainties could help loosen the grip of market fetishism on health professionals. Ambivalences are, after all, inherent in the attachments whereby we confront the otherwise unbearable "weight of the world" (Bourdieu 1999). Yet, the weight of the world can also be lessened.

My analysis of the medicalization of male circumcision in Turkey draws on in-depth research that includes interviews with circumcisers, families, and municipality employees, participant observation at circumcision settings, and archival research. This multimethod approach allowed me to investigate male circumcision as an ever-changing, dynamic, and multifaceted phenomenon embedded within broader institutional and organizational contexts shaped by national and global forces.

DEAUTHORIZING THE OFFICIAL NARRATIVE

To understand the historical transformation of male circumcision in Turkey, I examined newspaper articles, official local and national government documents, an unpublished memoir of a health officer, an educational book about medical circumcision written by another health officer, and scientific publications on male circumcision from the 1920s to the present. All these data enabled me to make sense of how male circumcision has been represented and discussed by those with cultural and political capital, such as medical professionals and government officials. A key finding was that the issue of male circumcision was entangled with the national elites' broader concerns about modernization, population, and social cohesion. Another finding was that these actors' narratives assumed a smooth transition from itinerant circumcisers to health officers and then to doctors. As medical actors introduced better circumcision techniques, the narrative suggests, actors with older techniques simply disappeared from the circumcision scene.

To deauthorize the official archive and narrative, I also established my own archive by conducting interviews with circumcisers. My interviews with sixty health officers indicated that the medicalization initiated by the medico-bureaucratic process was not always welcomed by families who operated with a nonmedical understanding of care. These opposing views sometimes created tension around what were acceptable forms of circumcision between families and health officers who wanted to educate families about medical techniques and take over the practice from itinerant circumcisions. The interviews, therefore, portrayed the medicalization of male circumcision as a negotiated space, rather than a top-down process, as is assumed by the official discourse on male circumcision.

Moreover, besides the tensions with families, health officers were generally silent about their conflicts with itinerant circumcisers. In this regard, my in-depth interviews with twenty itinerant circumcisers provided a richer account of the transition from traditional to scientific circumcision in the post–World War II period than what the official narrative presented. One of the crucial findings was that the transition was far from smooth and indeed rather conflict-ridden and violent. Itinerant circumcisers, most of whom performed circumcision illegally, recounted their troubles with the state authorities. The other finding was that while the official discourse interprets some families' resistance against medical techniques as a sign of ignorance, my interviews with itinerant circumcisers contradicted the official discourse: many families were not against the medical techniques but rather the health officers who represented the state. Juxtaposing the interviews with health officers and those with itinerant circumcisers enabled me to reveal the blind spots of the Turkish official discourse on male circumcision.

To conduct the interviews, I traveled to twenty-five cities and some of their outlying towns and villages and recruited my interviewees via snowball sampling. I was born and grew up in Istanbul and had not visited many of these places before embarking on my research. As a stranger, I would thus first go to a barbershop or a coffeehouse (kahvehane), the two popular settings where men socialize. Locals then directed me to circumcisers in their vicinities. If I could schedule all the interviews on the same day, then I moved on to my next stop (a new city, a town, or a village) without staying overnight. If not, I left the next day upon the completion of my interviews.

As the interviews proceeded, I reformulated new questions to broaden the scope of my data. For instance, my initial interviews revealed short-term collaborations between health officers and itinerant circumcisers, which was a surprising finding. I then added a question about such collaborations to the following interviews. While my interviews with health officers were recorded and transcribed, almost none of the itinerant circumcisers allowed me to record the interviews due to safety concerns. Some of those itinerant circumcisers gave consent to note-taking.

Being a male researcher had its advantages and disadvantages. I traveled to different regions of the country, often by bus and sometimes by plane, stayed at hotels, and visited male-dominated settings without concern for safety—a privilege that a female researcher would likely not have in Turkey. Homosocial

bonding practices also made it easy for me to establish rapport with my interviewees. For instance, some of my interviewees made jokes about penises and
shared what they considered funny and obscene stories with me. It would not
be far-fetched to assume that a female researcher would not have had such
intimate interactions with interviewees about male circumcision.

My gender identity presented obstacles too, though. Circumcisers sometimes found it strange that I as a Turkish man wanted to talk about male
circumcision: "Why do you want to talk about male circumcision? Aren't you
circumcised? You must already know all of this," some circumcisers asked. As a
response, I emphasized my intention to learn about their techniques and interactions with other circumcisers. I strategically presented myself as a stranger so
that my interviewees would not assume a shared cultural background between
us. For instance, I highlighted my affiliation with an American university and
the number of years I had been living abroad. Some circumcisers took these
facts as a sign of lacking cultural familiarity and even praised my Turkish
before providing some basic information about the ritual (for instance, how
celebrations are organized).

Moreover, some circumcisers were initially hesitant to talk to me because
they thought that I wanted to learn from them how to perform circumcision.
In their eyes, I was a man who was asking detailed questions about the operation: Where and how much do you apply local anesthesia? How long do you
wait before cutting off the foreskin? What instruments are you using? How do
you stitch the incision closed? They became suspicious of my intentions and
regarded me as a potential future competitor. As I discuss elsewhere (Başaran
2022), while I assured my informants about the purpose of my research, I
viewed their suspicion as an opportunity, rather than simply as an obstacle to
overcome, enabling me to understand the stakes of performing circumcision
in a competitive environment.

CIRCUMCISION FESTIVALS AND OPERATIONS

For my research, I also participated in circumcision events and operations for
four consecutive summers between 2011 and 2014, with additional short trips
between 2018 and 2021. I attended mass circumcision festivals organized by
municipalities in Istanbul and countless operations in different parts of the
country. These operations took place at hospitals, clinics, and homes. I gained
access to these settings through a variety of methods. The festivals were open
to the public, and I talked formally and informally with families at these
events. Almost all the elders, especially grandfathers, had been circumcised by
itinerant circumcisers in villages, and some of their sons had been circumcised

at mass circumcision events in cities in the 1970s and '80s. My dialogue with families thus provided a valuable comparative perspective on the divergent meanings attributed to male circumcision and the different ways male circumcision had been organized. Given the political significance of these events for municipalities, I also paid attention to the interactions between municipality employees and families and the ways in which municipalities have deployed the ritualistic aspect of male circumcision for political gains (for example, distributing gifts to boys). All these observations were recorded in field notes.

I accessed home-based operations through circumcisers. Either before or after the interviews with circumcisers, circumcisers put me in touch with families, and I got permission to attend the operations. The circumcisers and I went to families' homes, where boys were circumcised on a flat surface (often, on the floor). I did not take notes at the sites, as I was often asked to help the circumcisers and families with the operations. I sometimes held down the boys and verbally comforted them at other times. I shared with them the story of my circumcision. These moments were not merely an opportunity for me to immerse myself deeply in my research but also felt like a moral obligation to boys and their families, as I hoped that my support would make the operation less burdensome for them. My daily recorded observations about circumcisions carried out in homes focused on circumcisers' styles and techniques and their interactions with boys and their families.

Hospital managers and clinic owners granted me access to the medical settings in which most of the operations take place these days. At mass circumcisions, where the boys of low-income families were circumcised, I waited with families and talked to them informally about their sons' circumcisions and male circumcision in general. Some families invited me to watch the operations and others asked whether I could help their sons calm down before the operation or hold them down during the operation. Again, my goal was to pay attention to the ways mass operations were organized and carried out as well as the interactions between medical professionals (doctors and nurses) and families and between parents and their sons. After the completion of the operations, I interviewed the doctors who performed the operations. Doing so enabled me to understand mass circumcisions from different perspectives.

I frequented clinics serving middle-class families in Istanbul. Since circumcisions at these clinics were more efficient and better organized than mass circumcisions, I was never asked to be part of the operations for support. My formal and informal conversations with families and my observations of the interactions between families and circumcisers at these settings—interactions that were, contrary to mass circumcisions, (almost) devoid of tensions and conflicts—were crucial for my analysis of how class has shaped the experience of male circumcision. Each day I recorded and reviewed my field notes. I also interviewed the health officers who owned the clinics. These interviews, among other things, helped me to compare home-based circumcisions and clinic-based circumcisions from the perspective of circumcisers.

Finally, the emotional intensity of crossing different class settings during my research informed my analysis in chapters 4 and 5. I was moving back and forth between drastically different, even opposite atmospheres, sometimes on the same day: while I was very nervous and disturbed by boys' screams at mass circumcisions, my mood always noticeably changed when I entered the clinics. I was calm and relaxed. Although my own home-based circumcision was nothing like these mass circumcisions, the mass circumcisions nonetheless brought back memories of fear and postoperative pain. Reflecting on my emotions thus provided a basis for my analysis of the relationship between class, emotions, and male circumcision in contemporary Turkey.

NOTES

PROLOGUE

1. *Düğün*, in Turkish, literally translates as "wedding." However, it also refers to celebrations (sünnet düğünü) organized for circumcision, and "düğün salonu" is an indoor venue wherein many middle-class families organize these celebrations.

INTRODUCTION

1. To protect the anonymity of my informants, I use pseudonyms throughout the book.

2. Anatolia is the westernmost protrusion of Asia, which constitutes the majority of modern-day Turkey.

3. The relationship between psychoanalysis and sociology in the US (though certainly not in other parts of the world) has been weak since World War II, partly because of the positivist tendencies within US sociology and partly because of its anxiety over its status as a "science." For the history of US sociology's shifting attitude toward psychoanalysis, with examples of works that creatively bring together sociology and different psychoanalytical approaches, see Chancer and Andrews (2014).

4. For Freud, ambivalence is essential to the identification process. Ambivalence refers to unresolvable contradictory affective orientations toward the same object at once (not only tangible objects and people but also abstract ideas such as the nation); a combination of attraction to, and repulsion from, the object. Certain specific conflicts draw the attention of psychoanalysis, though: only those that "constitute a non-dialectical opposition which the subject, saying 'yes' and 'no' at the same time, is incapable of transcending" (Laplanche and Pontalis 1988, p. 28). A subject (a boy, in this case) within a family, Freud says, receives two conflicting messages: the directive "You ought to be like this (like your father)" is supplemented by a prohibition, "You may not be like this (like your father)," that is, "you may not do all that he does; some things are his prerogative" (Freud 1960, p. 30). The boy is enticed and demanded to behave like his father and at the same time taught that becoming like him might suggest a violation of a prohibition (and, more generally, of norms and prescriptions). The boy, in other words, asks, as French psychoanalyst Jacques Lacan puts it, a deeply troubling but fundamentally crucial question: *Che Vuoi?*—What does the Other want from me?—the

question that grounds the inauguration of the subject into a socio-symbolic order (Fink 1995).

5. I am using the notion of fantasy in a Lacanian sense: a scenario that constitutes and coordinates our desires. For the use of this concept of fantasy in nonclinical contexts, see Aretxaga (2003), Navaro-Yashin (2002a), and Žižek (1997).

6. Male circumcision is an ancient rite practiced by diverse communities, including ancient Egyptians, indigenous Australians, and indigenous inhabitants of southern Africa (see Anwer et al. 2017; Rizvi et al. 1999). The oldest accounts of male circumcision come from Egyptian tomb work and wall paintings dating from around 2300 BCE, and in the Semitic tradition (particularly, in Judaism and Islam), male circumcision is linked to a covenant with God dating back to Abraham (see Silverman 2006; Darby 2005). At present, an estimated 30 percent of males globally are circumcised, and two-thirds of these are Muslims (see Morris et al. 2016; WHO 2007). Hygiene, religion, ethnic and kinship bonds, and codes of masculinity are among the main reasons for male circumcision.

Religion is an important motivation behind male circumcision. Male circumcision is virtually universal in Jewish and Muslim populations. According to Judaism, circumcision emulates menstruation to "invest men with the ability to reproduce the community" (Silverman 2004, p. 424) and inscribes God's name onto boys' bodies. In a traditional Jewish circumcision, a baby is circumcised by a mohel on the eighth day after birth, in the presence of his family. In Islam, male circumcision is instead a recommended practice, as there is no specific mention of circumcision in the Quran. Islamic traditions, unlike Jewish circumcision traditions, do not include specific directions on the timing of the operation. Thus, the age of circumcision among Muslims varies based on, among other factors, region, nationality, and class, ranging from a few days after birth up to the age of eighteen. And circumcision in Turkish is simply known as *sunnah*, which refers to the traditions and practices of the Islamic prophet, Muhammad (Anwer et al. 2017; WHO 2007; Yegane et al. 2006).

Hygiene has been a crucial issue in the debates around male circumcision in Europe and the US. During the nineteenth century, male circumcision became increasingly popular in some English-speaking regions, especially in North America, as the medical community promoted the practice as a preventive measure (and sometimes punishment) for a range of conditions and behaviors including masturbation, syphilis, and bed-wetting (Aggleton 2007; Darby 2005). Nowadays, male circumcision in the US is typically performed soon after birth, as much for health-related reasons (such as preventing disease and infection) as for sociocultural reasons, including fathers' wishes to share a physical resemblance with their sons, parents' concerns regarding their sons' relationship to a future peer group, and parents' aesthetic preferences (Sardi and Livingston 2015; Mielke 2013; Binner et al. 2002; Tiemstra, 1999).

7. Male circumcision is also seen as a rite of passage to manhood in many other cultures across the world, including those of some sub-Saharan Africans, indigenous Australians, and inhabitants of the Philippines, eastern Indonesia, and various Pacific islands (WHO 2007). These rites are symbolically saturated with themes such as masculine

virility, fertility, opposition between men and women, preparation for marriage and adult sexuality, and blood sacrifice to the ancestors (Silverman 2004; Turner 1967; Bettelheim 1962). In some of these settings, male circumcision reproduces ethnic boundaries within a country in which one group is circumcised and the other one is not. Also, uncircumcised boys in settings where male circumcision is the cultural norm can face discrimination and punishment, including bullying and beatings (see, for instance, Vincent 2008). These rite-of-passage circumcisions are usually (but not always) performed when boys are older than the age of six (WHO 2007).

8. For instance, for the Xhosa of South Africa, talking about male circumcision in public is very much frowned upon (see Vincent 2008).

9. For a similar approach to female circumcision, see Hodžić (2017).

10. Sociologists and anthropologists have shown that medicalization is a stratified, contested, and negotiated process, as it relies on and generates different forms of inequalities (Clarke 2010). On the side of drivers of medicalization, it can empower and legitimize certain actors over others via regulations, laws, and codes (doctors over midwives, in the case of the medicalization of childbirth, or, as another example, a patent that grants exclusive rights to a company in the pharmaceutical market). On the side of laypeople, marginalized groups can be undermedicalized as they lack access to medical technologies and care and/or overmedicalized as they become subject to punitive techniques of surveillance and risk (Bridges 2011; Metzl 2010; Nelson 2011; Wailoo 2001). Constructions of race, gender, and class are implicated in scientific inquiries into the causes of the prevalence of certain diseases and illnesses among certain populations (Shim 2014; Shostak 2013).

11. See for instance Imber (2008).

12. Sociologists have analyzed ambivalences in a general sense as well. With some exceptions, such as Smelser (1998), ambivalences in classic and contemporary sociology have, however, largely been seen as either contingent or necessary byproducts of the social order and more specifically modernity and postmodernity. Robert Merton (1976), views ambivalences as resulting from conflicting social roles (for instance, being both a mother and a teacher) and argues for a sociological notion of ambivalence that, he believes, is fundamentally different from psychological ambivalence since the latter overlooks broader social forces. Another sociologist, Zygmunt Bauman (1991), inspired by a Derridean analysis of language and difference, conceptualizes ambivalences as an essential feature of the emergence of a social order based on oppositions such as friends and enemies. In this order, he argues, strangers occupy an ambiguous status embodying debilitating ambivalences that dualistic modern ideologies (for instance, nationalism) seek—ultimately unsuccessfully—to suppress because strangers blur the boundaries between friends and enemies. Similarly, Ulrich Beck (1994) and Anthony Giddens (1990) view ambivalences as a key aspect of (high) modernity. In contrast, I view ambivalence as a theoretical postulate rather than a historically contingent possibility: ambivalence is the inevitable consequence, and the condition of, our induction into socio-symbolic worlds.

13. For more on research methods, see appendix.

CHAPTER I: ITINERANT CIRCUMCISERS

1. In Turkish, *alaylı* refers to a person who has not been formally educated but learned a craft from his or her master, while *okullu*, the term that is occasionally used for health officers, refers to a person who has been formally educated.

2. As we shall see in the next chapter, health officers would change the standard circumcision position to having boys lie down on a flat surface in order to be able to use the medical techniques safely.

3. On classic patriarchy in the case of urban Egypt, see Inhorn (1996).

4. That classic patriarchy rests on the subordination of women should, however, not blind us to the various forms of negotiation carried out by women of all ages on a daily basis under this patriarchal structure (Sirman 1991). For an analysis of the persistence and transformation of classic patriarchal relations in urban areas in contemporary Turkey, see White (2004) and Sarıoğlu (2013).

5. The gendered classification of the public sphere existed elsewhere besides the rural areas where the majority of the population lived in the pre-1950s. In urban areas, up until the 1980s, urban middle-class married women's presence in public was very limited as well. Women who lived in modern apartment buildings were expected, ideally, to remain at home, and the male doorman (kapıcı) used to run many small errands, including grocery shopping (Ozyegin 2001).

6. *Kirve* is a term of a particular fictive kinship system called *kirvelik*. Kirvelik connects "two families or agnatic kin groups with prescribed duties, responsibilities and relations of gift and taboo in an exclusive relationship to descent and affinity. It, too, is usually established through ritual sponsorship, which in this case, especially in the contemporary context, generally involves sponsoring the Islamic rite of male circumcision" (Sengul 2014, p. 33).

7. See also Steinmetz (1999).

8. As in Europe (Emsley 1999), the gendarmerie (jandarma) has been essential to modern state formation in both the late Ottoman Empire and the Turkish Republic since the nineteenth century (Özbek 2008). The ruling elites aimed to extend their authority over provinces by charging gendarmerie with the tasks of maintaining order and security in provinces.

9. For more on this subject, see chapter 5.

10. Meyrankort grew in the region and was also believed to be beneficial for diabetes.

11. A common gesture to show respect to elder people of both genders in Turkey.

12. Chapter 3 will discuss in depth the tension between self-interest and altruism.

CHAPTER 2: FENNİ SÜNNETÇİ

1. Health professionals used catgut sutures for circumcision until the Turkish state banned them in 2008 in compliance with the EU public health rules. The rationale behind the prohibition was that these sutures used animal tissues or derivatives, increasing the risk of transmitting bovine spongiform encephalopathy (commonly known as "mad

cow disease"); despite being called "catgut," these sutures were usually manufactured from the intestines of goats or sheep. After the ban, the catgut sutures were mostly replaced with absorbable synthetic sutures. However, some health officers continued using catgut sutures and obtained them through informal networks.

2. The new state's relationship with Islam was selective and pragmatic. As in the case of France, which went beyond solely separating the state and the church, the Turkish state wanted to regulate religion by bringing it under its own control (Kuru 2009; Kadioğlu 1996). Accordingly, the state introduced such reforms as abolishing the office of the caliphate and religious courts; dissolving the dervish orders; granting women equal rights with men regarding divorce, inheritance, and child custody; and making free elementary education for both sexes mandatory.

3. In the 1930s, the child mortality rate was 27 percent of births, and the average life expectancy was thirty-five years. For those who survived the age of five, the average expectation of remaining life was fifty years (Günal 2008).

4. *Ülkü* was a journal that was published by the People's Houses between 1933 and 1950. These houses were opened to educate citizens according to modern-nation principles in the early years of the Republic (Öztürkmen 1994). The main contributors were politicians, historians, linguistics experts, and novelists.

5. The CHP (Republican People's Party), Turkey's oldest political party, was founded by the nationalist revolutionary leader Atatürk. The CHP was the nation's only party from 1923 to 1945.

6. Between 1963 and 1980, the number of health posts increased from 19 to 1,467, and the number of health stations increased from 37 to 5,776 (Günal 2008). The number of medical schools (Sağlık Koleji) for health officers increased from 1 to 9 between 1927 and 1960, and then to 37 during the period between 1960 and 1972 (TURKSTAT). Between 1960 and 1970, the number of health officers (who were exclusively men) increased from 3,550 to almost 10,000. Also, the ratio of population to health officer decreased from 13,072 to 3,810 between 1928 and 1980 (TURKSTAT). Moreover, the number of pharmacies in Turkey increased from 556 to 1,282 between 1949 and 1961 (http-//www.e-kutuphane.teb.org.tr/pdf/tebakademi/insan_gucu/7).

7. Some of my interviewees were already part of this infrastructure before the implementation of the developmentalist project.

8. Such a variety of responses to medicalization can be observed in colonial and postcolonial contexts. See Arnold (1993), Cosminsky (2016), Hunt (1999), and Lindenbaum and Lock (1993).

9. Abdals refer to an ethno-religious group known for performing circumcision and playing music at weddings and other events. See chapter 1. And *gypsy* in this context is a catchall derogatory term used for Abdals.

CHAPTER 3: MASS CIRCUMCISION

1. It is important to note that my analysis of the significance of mass imperial circumcisions for the Ottoman rule does not exhaust the broad range of meanings these

organizations had during the Ottoman Era. In general, the relationship between Muslim rulers and charitable activities has a long and rich history. These activities, for instance, were pious means for rulers to communicate with and please Allah and achieve redemption and salvation (Frenkel and Lev 2009). But this does not mean that the transcendent and sacred nature of charitable activities did not gain political and social functions in reproducing hierarchies and distinctions. The latter is the focus of this chapter.

2. Chapter 5 will demonstrate that this stigmatization gained a new impetus as political Islam in the 1990s began to consolidate its influence among the rural-to-urban population.

3. As chapter 5 will show, this is no longer the case for health officers in the neoliberal era.

4. Bourdieu was hesitant to embrace a psychoanalytical language. See Steinmetz (2006).

CHAPTER 4: FEAR OF CIRCUMCISION

1. See for instance Borrell-Carrió et al. (2004), Engel (1980), and Ghaemi (2010).

2. See for instance Good (1992) and Ware (1992).

3. See for instance Clark et al. (1999).

4. Here, I join Zeynep Korkman (2015a) and Sara Ahmed (2004) in bringing the nonconscious and conscious aspects of the experience and management of emotions into the same analytical focus.

5. https://www.dailymotion.com/video/x6x2lks; Özalp (n.d.).

6. See Arnould and Cayla (2015), Mazzarella (2003), Olsen (2020), and Schwarzkopf (2012).

7. One can contest the analytical value of the concept of the sovereign consumer for overlooking the fact that actual consumers face various constraints—including regulatory (for instance, state regulations on purchasing certain products), economic (not having enough disposable income), or logistical (information asymmetries) constraints. Indeed, over the last few decades, economic sociologists have successfully challenged mainstream economists' assumption about the ideal-typical market and market actors as self-interested actors who supposedly engage in one-time transactions based on full information. Markets are rather, they showed, always embedded within a socio-historical-cultural nexus (see, for instance, Wherry 2012; Zelizer 2011). The significance of this reservation notwithstanding, calling a fiction untrue does not make it disappear or eliminate its role in shaping social relations.

8. More details on his practice are shared later in this chapter.

9. Over the last few years, a new iteration of this script has emerged in Turkey: some mothers now wear their wedding dresses for their sons' circumcision celebrations. This strengthens the unresolved ambivalence central to male circumcisions and complicates the discussion in chapter 2 about whether circumcisions enact the separation of sons from their mothers. Or is circumcision another form of union between mothers and

now circumcised sons? This further attests to the fundamentally performative and fragile nature of masculinity.

10. For the relationship between the Turkish military and masculinity, see Açıksöz (2012).

CHAPTER 5: "DECEITFUL CHILD" AND "BAD PARENTS"

1. These hospitals are MLPCARE, ACIBADEM, Baskent Universitesi Hastaneleri, MEMORIAL, and MEDICANA.

2. To illustrate his point, Dr. Cengiz gave the example of hypospadias. Hypospadias refers to a condition in which the opening of the urethra is on the underside, rather than at the tip, of the penis. This birth defect can be identified only in medical examination, and babies with hypospadias should not be circumcised since the extra tissue of the foreskin may be needed to repair hypospadias in the future. Doctors also mentioned to me other medical conditions such as phimosis and paraphimosis that would escape the radar of health officers. While phimosis refers to the inability to retract the foreskin covering the glans of the uncircumcised penis, paraphimosis is a condition in which the retracted foreskin of the uncircumcised penis cannot be returned to its normal position, which may result in gangrene. In both cases, immediate attention is required and circumcision is recommended.

CONCLUSION

1. See the organization's website: https://www.intactamerica.org.

REFERENCES

Açıksöz, S. C. 2012. "Sacrificial Limbs of Sovereignty: Disabled Veterans, Masculinity, and Nationalist Politics in Turkey." *Medical Anthropology Quarterly* 26 (1): 4–25.

Açıksöz, S. C. 2015. "Ghosts Within: A Genealogy of War Trauma in Turkey." *Journal of the Ottoman and Turkish Studies Association* 2 (2): 259–280.

Adalet, B. 2018. *Hotels and Highways: The Construction of Modernization Theory in Cold War Turkey*. Redwood City, CA: Stanford University Press.

Agartan, T. I. 2015. "Health Workforce Policy and Turkey's Health Care Reform." *Health Policy* 119 (12): 1621–1626.

Aggleton, P. 2007. "'Just a Snip'?: A Social History of Male Circumcision." *Reproductive Health Matters* 15 (29): 15–21.

Ahmed, S. 2013. *The Cultural Politics of Emotion*. Oxfordshire, England: Routledge.

Aker, A. T., P. Önen, and H. Karakiliç. 2007. "Psychological Trauma: Research and Practice in Turkey." *International Journal of Mental Health* 36 (3): 38–57.

Aksakoğlu, G. 2008. "Sağlikta: Sosyalleştirmenin Öyküsü." *Memleket Siyaset Yönetim Dergisi*, no. 8, 7–62.

Anwer, A. W., L. Samad, S. Iftikhar, and N. Baig-Ansari. 2017. "Reported Male Circumcision Practices in a Muslim-Majority Setting." *BioMed Research International*, 2017.

Aran, M. A., and J. S. Hentschel. 2012. *Protection in Good and Bad Times? The Turkish Green Card Health Program*. Washington, DC: World Bank, Europe and Central Asia Region, Human Development Department.

Aretxaga, B. 2003. "Maddening States." *Annual Review of Anthropology* 32 (1): 393–410.

Arnold, D. 1993. *Colonizing the Body: State Medicine and Epidemic Disease in Nineteenth-Century India*. Oakland: University of California Press.

Arnould, E. J., and J. Cayla. 2015. "Consumer Fetish: Commercial Ethnography and the Sovereign Consumer." *Organization Studies* 36 (10): 1361–1386.

Artvinli, F. 2013. *Delilik, Siyaset ve Toplum: Toptaşı Bimarhanesi (1873–1927)*(Madness, politics, and society: The Toptaşı Asylum [1873–1927]). Istanbul: Boğaziçi University Press.

Aslan, S. 2015. *Governing Kurdish and Berber Dissent*. Cambridge, England: Cambridge University Press.

Aslan, S. 2009. "Incoherent State: The Controversy over Kurdish Naming in Turkey." *European Journal of Turkish Studies*, no. 10, 2–17.

175

Ataseven, A. 2005. *Tarih boyunca sünnet.* Boğaziçi Yayınları.

Ballard, K., and M. A. Elston. 2005. "Medicalisation: A Multi-dimensional Concept." *Social Theory & Health* 3 (3): 228–241.

Basaran, O. 2014. "'You Are Like a Virus': Dangerous Bodies and Military Medical Authority in Turkey." *Gender & Society* 28, no. 4 (August 2014): 562–582.

Başaran, O. 2021. "Neoliberalism, Welfare, and Mass Male Circumcisions in Turkey." *European Journal of Cultural and Political Sociology* 8 (1): 35–58.

Başaran, O. 2022. "In Praise of Suspicion." In *Silences, Neglected Feelings, and Blind-Spots in Research Practice*, 105–116. Oxfordshire, England: Routledge.

Bauman, Z. 1991. *Modernity and Ambivalence.* Ithaca, NY: Cornell University Press.

Beck, U. 1994. "The Reinvention of Politics: Towards a Theory of Reflexive Modernity." In *Reflexive Modernization: Politics, Tradition and Aesthetics in the Modern Social Order*, edited by Ulrich Beck, Anthony Giddens, and Scott Lash, 1–56. Redwood City, CA: Stanford University Press.

Bell, S. E., and A. E. Figert. 2012. "Medicalization and Pharmaceuticalization at the Intersections: Looking Backward, Sideways and Forward." *Social Science & Medicine* 75 (5): 775–783.

Benjamin, R. 2013. *People's Science: Bodies and Rights on the Stem Cell Frontier.* Redwood City, CA: Stanford University Press.

Berer, M. 2007. "Male Circumcision for HIV Prevention: Perspectives on Gender and Sexuality." *Reproductive Health Matters* 15 (29): 45–48.

Berlant, L. 2011. *Cruel Optimism.* Durham, NC: Duke University Press.

Bettelheim, B. 1962. *Symbolic Wounds: Puberty Rites and the Envious Male.* New, revised ed. New York: Collier Books.

Bhabha, H. K. 1994. *The Location of Culture.* Oxfordshire, England: Routledge.

Bilir, M. K., and F. Artvinli. 2021. "The History of Mental Health Policy in Turkey: Tradition, Transition and Transformation." *History of Psychiatry* 32 (1): 3–19.

Binner, S. L., J. M. Mastrobattista, M.-C. Day, L. S. Swaim, and M. Monga. 2002. "Effect of Parental Education on Decision-Making about Neonatal Circumcision." *Southern Medical Journal* 95 (4): 457–461.

Boon, J. A. 1995. "Circumscribing Circumcision/Uncircumcision: An Essay Amid the History of Difficult Description." In *Implicit Understandings: Observing, Reporting and Reflecting on the Encounters between Europeans and Other Peoples in the Early Modern Era*, 556–585. Cambridge, England: Cambridge University Press.

Borrell-Carrió, F., A. L. Suchman, and R. M. Epstein. 2004. "The Biopsychosocial Model 25 Years Later: Principles, Practice, and Scientific Inquiry." *Annals of Family Medicine* 2 (6): 576–582.

Bourdieu, P. 1996. *The Rules of Art: Genesis and Structure of the Literary Field.* Redwood City, CA: Stanford University Press.

Bourdieu, P. 1999. *The Weight of the World: Social Suffering in Contemporary Society.* Redwood City, CA: Stanford University Press.

Bourdieu, P. 2005. *The Social Structures of the Economy.* Polity.

Bourdieu, P., and L. J. D. Wacquant. 1992. *An Invitation to Reflexive Sociology.* Chicago, IL: University of Chicago Press.

Buğra, A. 2007. "Poverty and Citizenship: An Overview of the Social-Policy Environment in Republican Turkey." *International Journal of Middle East Studies* 39 (1): 33–52.

Buğra, A., and Keyder, Ç. 2006. "The Turkish Welfare Regime in Transformation." *Journal of European Social Policy* 16 (3): 211–228.

Bridges, K. M. 2011. *Reproducing Race: An Ethnography of Pregnancy as a Site of Racialization.* Oakland: University of California Press.

Brodwin, P. 2013. *Everyday Ethics: Voices from the Front Line of Community Psychiatry.* Oakland: University of California Press.

Broom, A., J. Broom, E. Kirby, and G. Scambler. 2017. "Nurses as Antibiotic Brokers: Institutionalized Praxis in the Hospital." *Qualitative Health Research* 27 (13): 1924–1935.

Broom, A., E. Kirby, A. F. Gibson, J. J. Post, and J. Broom. 2017. "Myth, Manners, and Medical Ritual: Defensive Medicine and the Fetish of Antibiotics." *Qualitative Health Research* 27 (13): 1994–2005.

Broom, D. H., and R. V. Woodward. 1996. "Medicalisation Reconsidered: Toward a Collaborative Approach to Care." *Sociology of Health & Illness* 18 (3): 357–378.

Buchbinder, M. 2015. *All in Your head: Making Sense of Pediatric Pain.* Oakland: University of California Press.

Cahill, H. 2001. "Male Appropriation and Medicalization of Childbirth: An Historical Analysis." *Journal of Advanced Nursing* 33 (3): 334–342.

Cansever, G. 1965. "Psychological Effects of Circumcision." *British Journal of Medical Psychology* 38 (4): 321–331.

Chambliss, D. F. 1996. *Beyond Caring: Hospitals, Nurses, and the Social Organization of Ethics.* Chicago, IL: University of Chicago Press.

Chancer, L., and J. Andrews, eds. 2014. *The Unhappy Divorce of Sociology and Psychoanalysis: Diverse Perspectives on the Psychosocial.* New York: Springer.

Clarke, A. E., ed. 2010. *Biomedicalization: Technoscience, Health, and Illness in the U.S.* Durham, NC: Duke University Press.

Clough, P. T. 2008. "The Affective Turn: Political Economy, Biomedia and Bodies." *Theory, Culture & Society* 25 (1): 1–22.

Collins, R. 2019. *The Credential Society: An Historical Sociology of Education and Stratification.* New York: Columbia University Press.

Conrad, P. 2005. "The Shifting Engines of Medicalization." *Journal of Health and Social Behavior* 46 (1): 3–14.

Conrad, P. 2007. *The Medicalization of Society: On the Transformation of Human Conditions into Treatable Disorders.* Baltimore, MD: Johns Hopkins University Press.

Conrad, P., and J. W. Schneider. 1980. *Deviance and Medicalization, from Badness to Sickness.* Maryland Heights, MO: Mosby.

Cosar, S., and M. Yegenoglu. 2009. "The Neoliberal Restructuring of Turkey's Social Security System." *Monthly Review* 60 (11): 36–49.

Cosminsky, S. 2016. *Midwives and Mothers: The Medicalization of Childbirth on a Guatemalan Plantation*. Austin: University of Texas Press.

Darby, R. 2005. *A Surgical Temptation: The Demonization of the Foreskin and the Rise of Circumcision in Britain*. Chicago, IL: University of Chicago Press.

Delaney, C. 1991. *The Seed and the Soil: Gender and Cosmology in Turkish Village Society*. Oakland: University of California Press.

Dickson, Kim E., Nhan T. Tran, Julia L. Samuelson, Emmanuel Njeuhmeli, Peter Cherutich, Bruce Dick, Tim Farley, Caroline Ryan, and Catherine A. Hankins. 2011. "Voluntary Medical Male Circumcision: A Framework Analysis of Policy and Program Implementation in Eastern and Southern Africa." *PLoS Medicine 8* (11): 1–13.

Dole, C. 2004. "In the Shadows of Medicine and Modernity: Medical Integration and Secular Histories of Religious Healing in Turkey." *Culture, Medicine and Psychiatry* 28 (3): 255–280.

Dole, C. 2012. *Healing Secular Life: Loss and Devotion in Modern Turkey*. Philadelphia: University of Pennsylvania Press.

Dole, C. 2015. "The House That Saddam Built: Protest and Psychiatry in Post-Disaster Turkey." *Journal of the Ottoman and Turkish Studies Association* 2 (2): 281–305.

Drash, M. 2019. "Circumcising Human Subjects: An Evaluation of Experimental Foreskin Amputation Using the Declaration of Helsinki." *Bioethics* 33 (3): 393–398.

Duden, B. 1993. *Disembodying Women: Perspectives on Pregnancy and the Unborn*. Cambridge, MA: Harvard University Press.

Earp, B. D. 2013. "The Ethics of Infant Male Circumcision." *Journal of Medical Ethics* 39 (7): 418–420.

Ehrenreich, B., and D. English. 2010. *Witches, Midwives, and Nurses: A History of Women Healers*. 2nd edition. Feminist Press at the City University of New York.

el-Sharkawy, Youssra. 2019. "Egyptian Anti-circumcision Group Calls for an End to 'Male Genital Mutilation.'" *Al-Monitor*. https://www.al-monitor.com /originals/2019/12/egyptians-dispute-necessity-of-circumcision.html.

Engel, G. L. 1980. "The Clinical Application of the Biopsychosocial Model." *The American Journal of Psychiatry* 137 (5): 535–544.

Epstein, S. 1995. "The Construction of Lay Expertise: AIDS Activism and the Forging of Credibility in the Reform of Clinical Trials." *Science, Technology, & Human Values* 20 (4): 408–437.

Erder, S. 1999. "Where Do You Hail From? Localism and Networks in Istanbul." In *Istanbul: Between the Global and the Local*. Lanham, MD: Rowman & Littlefield.

Erman, T. 2001. "The Politics of Squatter (Gecekondu) Studies in Turkey: The Changing Representations of Rural Migrants in the Academic Discourse." *Urban Studies* 38 (7): 983–1002.

Emsley, C. 1999. *Gendarmes and the State in Nineteenth-Century Europe*. Oxford, England: Oxford University Press.

Eyal, G. 2013. "For a Sociology of Expertise: The Social Origins of the Autism Epidemic." *American Journal of Sociology* 118 (4): 863–907.

Fassin, D. 2009. "Another Politics of Life Is Possible." *Theory, Culture & Society* 26 (5): 44–60.

Fink, B. 1995. *The Lacanian Subject: Between Language and Jouissance.* Princeton, NJ: Princeton University Press.

Fox, R. C. 1980. "The Evolution of Medical Uncertainty." *Milbank Quarterly* 58 (1): 1–49.

Freidson, E. (1970) 2017. *Professional Dominance: The Social Structure of Medical Care.* Oxfordshire, England: Routledge.

Frenkel, M., and Y. Lev. 2009. *Charity and Giving in Monotheistic Religions.* Berlin: Walter de Gruyter.

Freud, S. 1960. *The Ego and the Id.* Edited by J. Strachey. Translated by J. Riviere. New York: Norton and Company.

Gamble, V. . 1993. "A Legacy of Distrust: African Americans and Medical Research." Supplement, *American Journal of Preventive Medicine* 9 (6): 35.

Garenne, M., A. Giami, and C. Perrey. 2013. "Male Circumcision and HIV Control in Africa: Questioning Scientific Evidence and the Decision-Making Process." In *Global Health in Africa: Historical Perspectives on Disease Control*, 185–211. Ohio University Press.

Ghaemi, S. N. 2010. *The Rise and Fall of the Biopsychosocial Model: Reconciling Art and Science in Psychiatry.* Baltimore, MD: Johns Hopkins University Press.

Giddens, A. 1990. *The Consequences of Modernity.* Redwood City, CA: Stanford University Press.

Goffman, E. 1990. *The Presentation of Self in Everyday Life.* New York: Doubleday.

Good, B. 1994. *Medicine, Rationality, and Experience: An Anthropological Perspective.* Cambridge, England: Cambridge University Press.

Good, M.-J. D. 1992. *Pain as Human Experience: An Anthropological Perspective.* Oakland: University of California Press.

Gorman, E. H, and Sandefur, R. L. 2011. "'Golden Age,' Quiescence, and Revival: How the Sociology of Professions Became the Study of Knowledge-Based Work." *Work and Occupations* 38 (3): 275–302.

Günal, A. 2008. "Health and Citizenship in Republican Turkey: An Analysis of the Socialization of Health Services in Republican Historical Context." PhD diss., Istanbul: Boğazici Üniversitesi.

Herzfeld, M. 2004. *The Body Impolitic: Artisans and Artifice in the Global Hierarchy of Value.* Chicago, IL: University of Chicago Press.

Hochschild, A. R. 2012. *The Managed Heart: Commercialization of Human Feeling.* New edition with new preface. Oakland: University of California Press.

Hodžić, S. 2017. *The Twilight of Cutting: African Activism and Life after NGOs.* Oakland: University of California Press.

Humphrey, D. C. 1973. "Dissection and Discrimination: The Social Origins of

Cadavers in America, 1760–1915." *Bulletin of the New York Academy of Medicine* 49 (9): 819–827.

Hunt, N. R. 1999. *A Colonial Lexicon of Birth Ritual, Medicalization, and Mobility in the Congo.* Durham, NC: Duke University Press.

Illich, I. 1976. *Medical Nemesis: The Expropriation of Health.* New York: Pantheon Books.

Imber, J. B. 2008. *Trusting Doctors.* Princeton, NJ: Princeton University Press.

Inhorn, M. C. 1996. *Infertility and Patriarchy: The Cultural Politics of Gender and Family Life in Egypt.* Philadelphia: University of Pennsylvania Press.

Jerak-Zuiderent, S. 2012. "Certain Uncertainties: Modes of Patient Safety in Healthcare. *Social Studies of Science* 42 (5): 732–752.

Johnson, M. T. 2013. "Religious Circumcision, Invasive Rites, Neutrality and Equality: Bearing the Burdens and Consequences of Belief." *Journal of Medical Ethics* 39 (7): 450–455.

Joyce, K. A. 2008. *Magnetic Appeal: MRI and the Myth of Transparency.* Ithaca, NY: Cornell University Press.

Kadioğlu, A. 1996. "The Paradox of Turkish Nationalism and the Construction of Official Identity." *Middle Eastern Studies* 32 (2): 177–193.

Kandiyoti, D. 1998. "Bargaining with Patriarchy." *Gender and Society* 2 (3): 274–90.

Kandiyoti, D., and A. Saktanber, eds. 2002. *Fragments of Culture: The Everyday of Modern Turkey.* New Brunswick, NJ: Rutgers University Press.

Kapucu, N., and H. Palabıyık. 2008. *Turkish Public Administration: From Tradition to the Modern Age.* USAK Books.

Karakaya-Stump, A. 2018. "The AKP, Sectarianism, and the Alevis' Struggle for Equal Rights in Turkey." *National Identities* 20 (1): 53–67.

Karakaya-Stump, A. 2020. *Kizilbash-Alevis in Ottoman Anatolia: Sufism, Politics and Community.* Edinburgh, Scotland: Edinburgh University Press.

Katz, J. 1984. "Why Doctors Don't Disclose Uncertainty." *The Hastings Center Report* 14 (1): 35–44.

Kaufman, S. R. 1997. "Construction and Practice of Medical Responsibility: Dilemmas and Narratives from Geriatrics." *Culture, Medicine and Psychiatry* 21 (1): 1–26.

Kaufman, S. R. 2015. *Ordinary Medicine: Extraordinary Treatments, Longer Lives, and Where to Draw the Line.* Durham, NC: Duke University Press.

Kaya, D. G. 2015. "Coming to Terms with the Past: Rewriting History through a Therapeutic Public Discourse in Turkey." *International Journal of Middle East Studies* 47(4): 681–700.

Kayaoğlu, A., and S. Batur. 2013. "Critical Psychology in Turkey: Recent Developments." *Annual Review of Critical Psychology*, no. 10, 916–931.

Kırlı, C. 2004. "Coffeehouses: Public Opinion in the Nineteenth-Century Ottoman Empire." In *Public Islam and the Common Good,* 75–99. Brill.

Kleinman, A. 1980. *Patients and Healers in the Context of Culture: An Exploration of the Borderland between Anthropology, Medicine, and Psychiatry.* Oakland: University of California Press.

Kleinman, A. 1988. *The Illness Narratives: Suffering, Healing, and the Human Condition.* New York: Basic Books.

Kleinman, A. 2006. *What Really Matters: Living a Moral Life amidst Uncertainty and Danger.* Oxford, England: Oxford University Press.

Korkman, Z. K. 2015a. "Feeling Labor: Commercial Divination and Commodified Intimacy in Turkey." *Gender & Society* 29 (2): 195–218.

Korkman, Z. K. 2015b. "Fortunes for Sale: Cultural Politics and Commodification of Culture in Millennial Turkey." *European Journal of Cultural Studies* 18 (3): 319–338.

Kuru, A. T. 2009. *Secularism and State Policies toward Religion: The United States, France, and Turkey.* Cambridge, England: Cambridge University Press.

Lacan, J. 1997. *The Seminar of Jacques Lacan: The Ethics of Psychoanalysis 1959–1960.* Translated and annotated by Dennis Porter. New York: W. W. Norton.

Lambek, M. 2010. "Toward an Ethics of the Act." In *Ordinary Ethics: Anthropology, Language, and Action,* edited by M. Lambek, 1–39. New York, NY: Fordham University Press.

Langford, J. M. 2012. *Fluent Bodies: Ayurvedic Remedies for Postcolonial Imbalance.* Durham, NC: Duke University Press.

Laplanche, J., J. B. Pontalis, 1988. *Language of Psychoanalysis.* Translated by D. N. Smith. London: Karnac Books.

Latifoglu, O., R. Yavuzer, W. Ünal, A. Sari, S. Çenetoglu, and N. K. Baran. 1999. "Complications of Circumcision." *European Journal of Plastic Surgery* 22 (2): 85–88.

Lei, X. 2014. *Neither Donkey nor Horse: Medicine in the Struggle over China's Modernity.* Chicago, IL: University of Chicago Press.

Lewis, J. 1993. "Feminism, the Menopause and Hormone Replacement Therapy." *Feminist Review,* no. 43, 38–56.

Light, J. D. 1979. "Uncertainty and Control in Professional Training." *Journal of Health and Social Behavior* 20 (4): 310–322.

Lindenbaum, S., and M. M. Lock, eds. 1993. *Knowledge, Power, and Practice: The Anthropology of Medicine and Everyday Life.* Oakland: University of California Press.

Livne, R. 2019. *Values at the End of Life: The Logic of Palliative Care.* Cambridge, MA: Harvard University Press.

Loveman, M. 2005. "The Modern State and the Primitive Accumulation of Symbolic Power." *The American Journal of Sociology* 110 (6): 1651–1683.

Lupton, D. 1997. "Foucault and the Medicalisation Critique." In *Foucault, Health and Medicine,* edited by R. Bunton and A. Petersen. Oxfordshire, England: Routledge.

Mazor, J. 2013. "The Child's Interests and the Case for the Permissibility of Male Infant Circumcision." *Journal of Medical Ethics* 39 (7): 421–428.

Mazzarella, W. 2003. *Shoveling Smoke: Advertising and Globalization in Contemporary India.* Durham, NC: Duke University Press.

Mazzarella, W. 2017. *The Mana of Mass Society.* Chicago, IL: University of Chicago Press.

Merton, R. 1976. *Sociological Ambivalence and Other Essays.* New York: Free Press.

Metzl, J. M 2010. *The Protest Psychosis: How Schizophrenia Became a Black Disease.* Boston, MA: Beacon Press.

Mielke, R. T. 2013. "Counseling Parents Who Are Considering Newborn Male Circumcision." *Journal of Midwifery & Women's Health* 58 (6): 671–682. https://doi .org/10.1111/jmwh.12130.

Ministry of Health of Turkey. 2008. "Health Statistics Yearbook." https://www.saglik .gov.tr/TR,11647/saglik-arastirmalari-genel-mudurlugu-saglik-istatistikleri -yilligi-2008.html.

Ministry of Health of Turkey. 2010. "Health Statistics Yearbook." https://www.saglik .gov.tr/TR,11650/saglik-arastirmalari-genel-mudurlugu-saglik-istatistikleri -yilligi-2010.html.

Ministry of Health of Turkey. 2014. "Health Statistics Yearbook." http://saglik.gov.tr /TR/dosya/1-101702/h/yilliktr.pdf.

Ministry of Health of Turkey. 2019. "Health Statistics Yearbook." https://dosyasb .saglik.gov.tr/Eklenti/40566,health-statistics-yearbook-2019pdf.pdf?0.

Mol, A. 2008. *The Logic of Care: Health and the Problem of Patient Choice.* Oxfordshire, England: Routledge.

Morande, B. S. 2019. *Salud Callejera: Mobilizing Cuidado at the Margins of Neoliberalism, Reimagining Care for People Experiencing Homelessness in Buenos Aires.* Honors project, Bowdoin College. https://core.ac.uk/download/pdf/214030269.pdf.

Morris, B. J., R. G. Wamai, E. B. Henebeng, A. A. Tobian, J. D. Klausner, J. Banerjee, and C. A. 2016. "Estimation of Country-Specific and Global Prevalence of Male Circumcision." *Population Health Metrics* 14 (1): 1–13.

Navaro-Yashin, Y. 2002a. *Faces of the State: Secularism and Public Life in Turkey.* Princeton, NJ: Princeton University Press.

Navaro-Yashin, Y. 2002b. "The Market for Identities: Secularism, Islamism, Commodities." In *Fragments of culture: The everyday of modern Turkey*, edited by D. Kandiyoti and A. Saktanber, 221–254. New Brunswick, NJ: Rutgers University Press.

Nichter, M. 1998. "The Mission within the Madness: Self-Initiated Medicalization as Expression of Agency." In *Pragmatic Women and Body Politics*, edited by Margaret M. Lock and Patricia A. Kaufert, 327–354. Cambridge, England: Cambridge University Press.

Olsen, N. 2020. "Ludwig von Mises, the Idea of Consumer Democracy and the Invention of Neoliberalism." *The Tocqueville Review* 41 (2): 43–64.

Özalp, Alanur. n.d. "Çocuklarda Sünnet." Accessed May 17, 2022. http://www .alopsikolog.net/kose_bcep28.asp.

Özbay, F. 1995. "Changes in Women's Activities both Inside and Outside the Home." In *Women in Modern Turkish Society*, 89–111. London: Zed Books.

Özbek, N. 2008. "The Politics of Modern Welfare Institutions in the Late Ottoman Empire (1876–1909)." *International Journal of Turcologia* 3 (5): 42–62.

Özdemir, E. 1997. "Significantly Increased Complication Risks with Mass Circumcisions." *British Journal of Urology* 80 (1): 136.

Ozyegin, G. 2001. *Untidy Gender: Domestic Service in Turkey*. Philadelphia, PA: Temple University Press.

Özden, B. A. 2014. "The Transformation of Social Welfare and Politics in Turkey: A Successful Convergence of Neoliberalism and Populism." In *Turkey Reframed: Constituting Neoliberal Hegemony*, 157–174. Pluto Press.

Ozturk, O. M. 1973. "Ritual Circumcision and Castration Anxiety." *Psychiatry* 36 (1): 49–60.

Öztürkmen, A. 1994. "The Role of People's Houses in the Making of National Culture in Turkey." *New Perspectives on Turkey*, no. 11, 159–181.

Özyürek, E. 2006. *Nostalgia for the Modern: State Secularism and Everyday Politics in Turkey*. Durham, NC: Duke University Press.

Petryna, A. 2009. *When Experiments Travel: Clinical Trials and the Global Search for Human Subjects*. Princeton, NJ: Princeton University Press.

Polanyi, K. 2001. *The Great Transformation: The Political and Economic Origins of Our Time*. 2nd edition, paperback. Boston, MA: Beacon Press.

Rahimi, B. 2014. "Nahils, Circumcision Rituals and the Theatre State." In *Ottoman Tulips, Ottoman Coffee: Leisure and Lifestyle in the Eighteenth Century*, edited by D. Sajdi, 90–117. London: IB Tauris.

Reich, A. D. 2014. *Selling Our Souls: The Commodification of Hospital Care in the United States*. Princeton, NJ: Princeton University Press.

Rizvi, S. A. H., S. A. A. Naqvi, M. Hussain, and A. S. Hasan. 1999. "Religious Circumcision: A Muslim View." *BJU International* 83 (1): 13–16.

Rose, N. S. 1996. *Inventing Our Selves: Psychology, Power, and Personhood*. Cambridge, England: Cambridge University Press.

Sabah. 2013. "Sünnetçiler Artık Tarih Oluyor." Accessed May 17, 2022. https://www.sabah.com.tr/saglik/2013/06/21/sunnetciler-artik-tarih-oluyor.

Santner, E. L. 2001. *On the Psychotheology of Everyday Life: Reflections on Freud and Rosenzweig*. Chicago, IL: University of Chicago Press.

Sardi, L., and K. Livingston. 2015. "Parental Decision Making in Male Circumcision." *MCN, the American Journal of Maternal Child Nursing* 40 (2): 110–115.

Sari, N., S. C. Büyükünal, and B. Zülfikar. 1996. "Circumcision Ceremonies at the Ottoman Palace." *Journal of Pediatric Surgery* 31 (7): 920–924.

Sarıoğlu, E. 2013. "Gendering the Organization of Home-Based Work in Turkey: Classical versus Familial Patriarchy: Gendering the Organization of Home-Based Work in Turkey." *Gender, Work & Organization* 20, no. 5 (September 2013): 479–497.

Scheper-Hughes, N. 1992. *Death without Weeping: The violence of Everyday Life in Brazil*. Oakland: University of California Press.

Schutz, A. 1967. *The Phenomenology of the Social World*. Evanston, IL: Northwestern University Press.

Schwarzkopf, S. 2012. "The Market Order as Metaphysical Loot: Theology and the Contested Legitimacy of Consumer Capitalism." *Organization* 19 (3): 281–297.

Sengul, S. R. 2014. "Broken (His)tories inside Restored Walls: Kurds, Armenians and the Cultural Politics of Reconstruction in Urban Diyarbakir, Turkey." Phd diss., University of Texas at Austin.

Shim, J. K. 2014. *Heart-Sick: The Politics of Risk, Inequality, and Heart Disease.* New York, NY: New York University Press.

Shorter, F. C. 1985. "The Population of Turkey after the War of Independence." *International Journal of Middle East Studies* 17 (4): 417–441.

Shostak, S. 2013. *Exposed Science: Genes, the Environment, and the Politics of Population Health.* Oakland: University of California Press.

Silverman, E. K. 2004. "Anthropology and Circumcision." *Annual Review of Anthropology* 33 (1): 419–445.

Silverman, E. K. 2006. *From Abraham to America: A History of Jewish Circumcision.* Lanham, MD: Rowman & Littlefield.

Silverstein, B. 2003. "Islam and Modernity in Turkey: Power, Tradition and Historicity in the European Provinces of the Muslim World." *Anthropological Quarterly* 76, (3): 497–517.

Sirman, N. 1991. "Friend or Foe? Forging Alliances with Other Women in a Village of Western Turkey." In *Women in Modern Turkish Society.* London: Zed Books.

Smelser, N. J. 1998. "The Rational and the Ambivalent in the Social Sciences." *American Sociological Review* 63: 1–16.

Steinmetz, G., ed. 1999. *State/Culture: State-Formation after the Cultural Turn.* Ithaca, NY: Cornell University Press.

Steinmetz, G. 2006. "Bourdieu's Disavowal of Lacan: Psychoanalytic Theory and the Concepts of 'Habitus' and 'Symbolic Capital.'" *Constellations* 13 (4): 445–464.

Steinmetz, G. 2007. *The Devil's Handwriting: Precoloniality and the German Colonial State in Qingdao, Samoa, and Southwest Africa.* Chicago, IL: University of Chicago Press.

Szasz, T. 2007. *The Medicalization of Everyday Life: Selected Essays.* Syracuse, NY: Syracuse University Press.

Taussig, M. T. 1980. "Reification and the Consciousness of the Patient." *Social Science & Medicine. Part B: Medical Anthropology* 14 (1): 3–13.

Terzioglu, D. 1995. "The Imperial Circumcision Festival of 1582: An Interpretation." *Muqarnas, no.* 12, 84–100.

Tiemstra, J. D. 1999. "Factors Affecting the Circumcision Decision." *Journal of the American Board of Family Medicine* 12 (1): 16–20. https://doi.org/10.3122 /15572625-12-1-16.

Timmermans, S. 1998. "Social Death as Self-fulfilling Prophecy." *Sociological Quarterly* 39 (3): 453–472.

Timmermans, S., and A. Angell. 2001. "Evidence-Based Medicine, Clinical Uncertainty, and Learning to Doctor." *Journal of Health and Social Behavior* 42 (4): 342–359.

Timmermans, S., and Hyeyoung O. 2010. "The Continued Social Transformation of the Medical Profession." Supplement, *Journal of Health and Social Behavior* 51, no. 1 (2010): S94–106.

Topal, O. F. 2020. "The Politics of Male Circumcision in the Late Ottoman Empire." *Middle Eastern Studies* 57 (1): 1–13.

Topuzlu, C. 1935. *Sünnet Sağlık İçin Faydalı mıdır?* Istanbul: Akşam Matbaası.

TURKSTAT (Turkish Statistical Institute) (2006). *Statistical Indicators, 1923-2004.* TURKSTAT.

Turner, V. W. 1967. *The Forest of Symbols: Aspects of Ndembu Ritual.* Ithaca, NY: Cornell University Press.

Vincent, L. 2008. "'Boys will be boys': Traditional Xhosa Male Circumcision, HIV and Sexual Socialisation in Contemporary South Africa." *Culture, Health & Sexuality* 10 (5): 431–446.

Wacquant, L. J. D. 2004. *Body and Soul: Notebooks of an Apprentice Boxer.* Oxford, England: Oxford University Press.

Wailoo, K. 2001. *Dying in the City of the Blues: Sickle Cell Anemia and the Politics of Race and Health.* Chapel Hill: University of North Carolina Press.

Ware, N. C. 1992. "Suffering and the Social Construction of Illness: The Delegitimation of Illness Experience in Chronic Fatigue Syndrome." *Medical Anthropology Quarterly,* 6 (4), 347–361.

Warhurst, C., and D. Nickson. 2007. "Employee Experience of Aesthetic Labour in Retail and Hospitality." *Work, Employment and Society* 21 (1): 103–120.

Weber, M., H. Gerth, and C. W. Mills. 1946. *From Max Weber: Essays in Sociology.* Oxford, England: Oxford University Press.

Wherry, F. F. 2012. *The Culture of Markets.* Cambridge, England: Polity.

White, J. B. 2004. *Money Makes Us Relatives: Women's Labor in Urban Turkey.* Oxfordshire, England: Routledge.

WHO. 2007. *Neonatal and Child Male Circumcision: A Global Review.* https://www .malecircumcision.org/resource/neonatal-and-child-male-circumcision-global -review.

Yegane, R.-A., A.-R. Kheirollahi, N.-A. Salehi, M. Bashashati, J.-A. Khoshdel, and M. Ahmadi. 2006. "Late Complications of Circumcision in Iran." *Pediatric Surgery International* 22 (5): 442–445.

Yeğen, M. 1999. "The Kurdish Question in Turkish State Discourse." *Journal of Contemporary History* 34 (4): 555–568.

Yilmaz, M. 2015. "Türkiye' de kirsal nüfusun değişimi ve ilere göre dağilimi (1980–2012)." *Doğu Coğrafya Dergisi* 20 (33): 161–188.

Yılmaz, S. 2019. "Becoming Rıza Nur: Selfhood, Desire, and Memory in Hayatım ve Hatıratım." Paper presented at MESA (Middle East Studies Association), New Orleans, LA, November 14.

Yılmaz, V. 2017. *The Politics of Healthcare Reform in Turkey.* London: Palgrave Macmillan.

Yoltar, Ç. 2020. "Making the Indebted Citizen: An Inquiry into State Benevolence in Turkey." *Political and Legal Anthropology Review* 43 (1): 153–171.

Zelizer, V. A. R. 2005. *The Purchase of Intimacy*. Princeton, NJ: Princeton University Press.

Zelizer, V. A. R. 2011. *Economic Lives: How Culture Shapes the Economy*. Princeton, NJ: Princeton University Press.

Žižek, S. 1997. *The Plague of Fantasies*. London: Verso.

Zola, I. K. 1972. "Medicine as an Institution of Social Control." *The Sociological Review* 20 (4): 487–504.

INDEX

Photos and tables are indicated by italicized page numbers.

187

in medicalization, 7, 19, 24–25, 27, 43, 51; replacement of itinerant circumcisers, 7, 46, 49–52, 62–63, 67, 72, 76, 79; stigmatization and, 51–52, 76, 135; training and, 44, 71–73, 95

health officers, mass circumcisions and, 160; appointment system in, 102–104; performing, 77, 80–81, 87, 92–98, 131, 135, 137, 152; risks in, 99–102, 104, 135; training in, 95–97, 102

hemophilia, 133–134

herbs, 40–41, 171n10

Herzfeld, Michael, 32

HIV, 155

homosocial bonding practices, 5

honor code, 30

hospitals, 77, 149, 153; under AKP, 132, 136–138, 151–152, 159–160, 174n1; appointment system in, 20, 139; competition among, 137–138; families in, 141–146, 148; in neoliberalism, 21, 84; poor and, 132, 137–144, 148, 160; private, 17, 20, 132–136, 174n1; public, 138; trauma-based model in, 131

hostile worlds, 105

humor, in medical settings, 13

hygiene, 5, 169n6

hypospadias, 134, 174n2

Iceland, 155

identification, 75–76

ideology, 139; ambivalence and, 151, 155, 161, 170n12; Bad Parents, Deceitful Child in, 20, 131, 145–146, 151; doctors and, 20, 77, 131, 145–146, 160; mass circumcisions and, 20, 131, 145–146, 150–151, 160; nationalist, 55, 61; Westernization and, 57–58

iğneci (female healers), 67

imperial circumcision festivals, 81–84, 95

inequality: ethics and, 160–161; health officers and, 81, 104; male circumcision debate and, 155, 158, 161–162; mass circumcisions and, 8, 81, 104, 106; medicalization and, 15, 106, 170n10; subjectivity and, 8–9, 14, 106; welfare and, 85–86. See also class

institutionalization, mental health, 111

Intact America, 155

interpellation, 3, 10–11

interpretivism, 11–13

Islam: Alevis, 25–26; in early Turkish Republic, 53, 56–57, 173n2; male circumcision and, 155, 169n6; mass circumcisions and, 172n1; in Ottoman Empire, 83, 172n1; political, 87, 137, 173n2; sacrifice in, 101–102, 147; Sunni, 25, 57, 83

itinerant circumcisers, 21, 62–63, 79, 107, 149; Abdals, 23–27, 37–38, 49, 61, 67–68, 172n9; as alaylı, 24, 171n1; ambivalence of, 24, 32–33, 47; apprenticeship of, 24–26, 28–33; barbers, 26–27, 30–31, 42–43, 45, 65, 74–75, 91, 94; calculation and, 89–91; in Central Anatolia, 1, 23–24, 31, 37–38, 65; in classic patriarchy, 27–34; developmentalism and, 7–8, 19, 33–34; dispossession of, 7–8, 34–40, 76; doctors and, 48, 135; in early Turkish Republic, 1, 24, 33–35, 46, 55, 58; on hemophilia, 133–134; herbs used by, 40–41, 171n10; identification and, 75–76; in Kurdish region, 39–41; licenses for, 34–35, 73; local anesthesia and, 42–45, 50–51, 94; mass circumcisions and, 87, 135; medicalization discourse dismissing,